The New Leadership Challenge:

Creating the Future of Nursing

Sheila C. Grossman, PhD, APRN

Associate Professor
School of Nursing
Fairfield University
Fairfield, Connecticut

Theresa M. Valiga, EdD, RN

Director of Research and
Professional Development
National League for Nursing
New York, New York

 F. A. DAVIS COMPANY • Philadelphia

F. A. Davis Company
1915 Arch Street
Philadelphia, PA 19103

Printed in the United States of America

Last digit indicates print number: 10 9 8 7 6 5 4 3 2 1

Managing Publisher: Lisa A. Biello
Acquisitions Editor: Joanne P. DaCunha, RN, MSN
Developmental Editor: Diane Schweisguth, RN, BSN
Cover Designer: Louis J. Forgione

As new scientific information becomes available through basic and clinical research, recommended treatments and drug therapies undergo changes. The author(s) and publisher have done everything possible to make this book accurate, up to date, and in accord with accepted standards at the time of publication. The authors, editors, and publisher are not responsible for errors or omissions or for consequences from application of the book, and make no warranty, expressed or implied, in regard to the contents of the book. Any practice described in this book should be applied by the reader in accordance with professional standards of care used in regard to the unique circumstances that may apply in each situation. The reader is advised always to check product information (package inserts) for changes and new information regarding dose and contraindications before administering any drug. Caution is especially urged when using new or infrequently ordered drugs.

Library of Congress Cataloging-in-Publication Data

Grossman, Sheila.
    The new leadership challenge : creating the future of nursing / Sheila C. Grossman,
  Theresa M. Valiga.
        p. ; cm
    Includes bibliographical references and index.
    ISBN 0-8036-0594-3
    1. Nursing services—Administration. 2. Leadership. I. Valiga, Theresa M. II. Title.
  [DNLM: 1. Nursing, Supervisory. 2. Leadership. 3. Nurse Administrators. WY 105
  G8785n 1999]
  RT89.G77   1999
  362.1'73'068—dc21
                                                                                        99-042955

Author Biographies

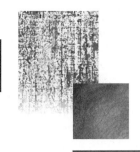

Sheila C. Grossman, PhD, APRN, received her baccalaureate degree in nursing and her doctoral degree in higher education professional administration from the University of Connecticut, and her master's degree from the University of Massachusetts in biophysiological nursing with a clinical nurse specialty in respiratory nursing. She has been a staff and charge nurse on a variety of medical-surgical units and intensive care units. She has been a critical care nursing instructor at Hartford Hospital and St. Francis Hospital and Medical Center, both in Hartford, CT. She has taught nursing at the University of Connecticut and currently is an Associate Professor in the School of Nursing at Fairfield University (CT), affiliating clinically at the Yale New Haven Hospital. Dr. Grossman has done multiple national and local presentations and publications in the areas of clinical decision making, critical care nursing outcome studies, leadership, and evidence-based practice. She is a past member of the Connecticut State Board of Nursing and a long-time active member of her local chapter of Sigma Theta Tau International and the American Association of Critical Care Nurses. She has recently completed her postmaster's certificate in advanced practice as a Family Nurse Practitioner.

Theresa M. Valiga, EdD, RN, received her bachelor's degree in nursing from Trenton State College (now The College of New Jersey) and her master's and doctoral degrees, both in nursing education, from Teachers College, Columbia University. She has been a faculty member at Trenton State College, Georgetown University, Seton Hall University, Villanova University, and Fairfield University, where she served as Dean of the School of Nursing. At present, she is the Director of Research and Professional Development at the National League for Nursing. Dr. Valiga's primary research interests relate to students' cognitive/intellectual development, critical thinking, and leadership development. Her publications, presentations, and consultations center around these topics, as well as curriculum development, creative teaching strategies, and various professional issues. She is the author of several articles and has coauthored two books: *The Nurse*

Educator in Academe: Strategies for Success and Using the Arts and Humanities to Teach Nursing: A Creative Approach. She recently served as Vice President of Sigma Theta Tau International and serves as National Vice President of the Interdisciplinary Honor Society of Phi Kappa Phi, and she has held numerous leadership positions in nursing throughout her career. Dr. Valiga also is the recipient of several awards, including the National League for Nursing Council of Constituent Leagues Leadership Award, the Sigma Theta Tau International Founders Award for Excellence in Education, and the National League for Nursing Isabel Stewart Award for Excellence in Nursing Education.

Reviewers

Connie J. Boerst, MSN, RN, C
Nursing Faculty
Bellin College of Nursing
Green Bay, Wisconsin

Mary L. Fisher, RN, PhD, CNNA
Associate Professor and Graduate
Curriculum Coordinator
Indiana University
Indianapolis, Indiana

Maryann F. Fralic, RN, DrPH, FAAN
Professor
School of Nursing
The Johns Hopkins University
Baltimore, Maryland

Ann Haffer, RN, MSN, EdD
Professor
California State University,
Sacramento
Division of Nursing
Sacramento, California

Barbara Jones, RN, DNSc
Associate Professor
Gwynedd Mercy College
Gwynedd Valley, Pennsylvania

Giovanna B. Morton, RN, EdD
Associate Dean/Professor
School of Nursing
Marshall University
Huntington, West Virginia

Edwin W. Schaefer, RN, ND
Instructor
Rush University
Chicago, Illinois

Donna Trainor, RN, EdD
Associate Professor
Massachusetts College of
Pharmacy and Allied Health
Boston, Massachusetts

Dedication

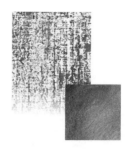

This book is dedicated to each and every nurse who is leading the profession to a preferred future and to my students, patients, mentors, and colleagues who have taught me so much about staying committed to a vision of enhancing leadership and followership. Also, I want to thank my husband, Bob; my daughters, Lisa and Beth; and my parents, sister, and brother, who have always inspired me to keep on task and do my best.

SG

This book is dedicated to the many faculty colleagues and hundreds of students I have known who have helped me crystallize my thinking about leadership and who, themselves, have taken on the challenge of providing leadership. Through dialogs in the classroom, papers that have been written, conversations in each other's offices, sharing of resources and ideas, and observing these individuals functioning as leaders, I have come to understand more fully the true meaning of what it means to be a leader. I also dedicate this book to my husband, Bob, who continues to support me in all my professional pursuits and whose patience and understanding have meant the world to me. Finally, I dedicate this book to my mother and father. Although neither of them is here to see its publication, they were a tremendous influence in my development as a professional and, hopefully, a leader; for that and for all they have given me, I will be forever grateful.

TV

Acknowledgments

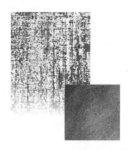

The authors wish to thank Joanne DaCunha for inviting us to explore the concept of leadership through a textbook and for her innovative ideas about what this book could be. We will always be grateful for her inspiration, her faith in us, and her ongoing support throughout the project. We also wish to extend our most heartfelt thanks to our production assistant, Diane Schweisguth. Her patience, feedback, suggestions, and guidance helped us write a book of which we are proud—a book we think can be extremely valuable to the nursing community.

Our gratitude also is extended to Dr. Melanie Dreher for her thoughtful reflections in the Foreword to this book and to Deborah Miles, MSN, APRN, for her input regarding quotes about leaders and leadership. Finally, we thank our families and friends for their love and support throughout the process of developing and writing this book.

Foreword

Why is leadership such an issue in nursing anyway? The significance of leadership in nursing is not new. Nursing, more than any other health profession, always has been practiced in an organizational context. The responsibility for unrelenting vigilance of patients typically and necessarily requires several nurses, one of whom generally emerges or is appointed as being "in charge." As a profession, we have embraced organizational theory, explored new management strategies, and learned the language of administration in both education and practice.

Until recently, much of our leadership has been inwardly focused, and we have done a good job at organizing ourselves. But with the exception of luminaries such as Florence Nightingale or Lillian Wald, our demonstrations of leadership have centered primarily on administration and on professional, rather than public, issues. As Drs. Grossman and Valiga so elegantly point out, however, leadership for the future implies not only organizational leadership but personal leadership and the exhibition of qualities that are deployed to improve patient care and reshape healthcare systems. It is not, as many would think, peripheral to "real" nursing—applicable only to managers and administrators. Rather, leadership is intrinsic to our advocacy roles with patients; to promoting healthier lifestyles for individuals, families, and communities; and to designing better healthcare systems. Nurses must understand how to lead in order to understand how to nurse.

Yet leadership is perhaps one of the most elusive concepts that guide nursing education. There is no single definition that encompasses all its many aspects. Furthermore, no one sets out to be a "leader." If we were to ask children what they would like to be when they are older, it would be highly unlikely that any would say, "I'm going to be a leader when I grow up." Even most leaders would not use the term "leader" to describe themselves. Rather, it is a term that others assign to an individual by virtue of his or her influence.

Despite its elusiveness, the concept of leadership is fundamental to nursing and somehow must be taught and learned. So how do we prepare students of nursing and neophyte clinicians to be leaders? In this fine and futuristic book, Drs. Grossman and Valiga assist students, faculty, and nurses in practice to deal with this dilemma by guiding their readers through the many dimensions of leadership. Through their carefully articulated objectives and exercises, they make the abstract concrete and the elusive tangible. They bring the future into the present and make the relationship between leadership and followership intelligible.

Significantly, this book takes leadership out of the domain of merely listing personal attributes or innate abilities and shows us how this elusive concept can be taught and learned. Leadership is not about power, but rather about acting powerfully. And leadership is not just about personal skill development such as assertiveness training, public speaking, or persuasive writing. Although there are some tools that prepare us to be more effective leaders, the essential motivation for leaderships lies in our commitment to the values we hold regarding a healthy and honorable society. Leadership is, however, about identifying social need and then mobilizing and configuring the intellectual and social capital to address that need. Leadership emerges when we are faced with a problem that is so compelling that we are obliged to take the risks we might not ordinarily take.

Drs. Grossman and Valiga show us that leadership is a lifetime undertaking that will take different forms throughout our careers. As we move into the future as a community of nursing scholars—occupying roles as clinicians, educators, researchers, and administrators—leadership development is essential to helping us realize the potential for greatness in each of us and in all of us. The future will require each of us to seize opportunities to express leadership, and this book helps prepare us for those challenges.

This volume acknowledges the difficulty in conceptualizing leadership and the fact that it often is easier to say what it is not than to say what it is. Thus, a theme that is both explicit and implicit in this volume—that of distinguishing leadership from management—holds great promise for helping students and nurses in practice to understand the essence of leadership. The authors do not equate being a dean or nurse executive or even a politician with being a leader. Although we hope that one gets into positions of influence because he or she has demonstrated some capacity for leadership along the way, we know this is not always the case.

Another consistent theme throughout this book is that leadership for the future needs to be about creating an environment in which expressions of leadership can flourish. Assuming any leadership role means substantial risk-taking, and the self-esteem and confidence required to take such risks almost always is derived externally from supporters; leaders for the future must not only assume leadership positions themselves, they also must nourish leadership in others. The authors' approach to followership and the importance of buttressing those who must agonize over the correctness and costs of controversial decisions is critical for understanding and promoting leadership.

Given the unparalleled advances in technology that the future will continue to bring, the emphasis on leadership, creativity, and innovation will be as important as knowledge. The relationship between vision and creativity in the generation and ongoing development of leaders, therefore, is critical, as these authors note.

At the same time that we are modeling leadership and exposing our students and nurses to leadership, we must identify leadership potential in young nurses and encourage them, mentor them. Our students and neophyte clinicians need to know this side of faculty and more experienced colleagues. They need to see us participating in public service and thinking freely. We need to do this not only for ourselves, but for them as well. The lack of commitment to public service and the absence of statespersonship in our society are lamentable. We can begin to change this state of affairs and exercise leadership ourselves when we teach our students and colleagues the value of public service—of making a commitment that goes beyond family and household and profession into society, indeed, into a global society.

The future is moving nursing, incontrovertibly, into the public arena. In the traditions of Nightingale and Wald, nursing once again is or will be at the forefront of social change, and the extent to which nurses address the problems of society will be the measure of our leadership. It is increasingly apparent that high-quality, accessible, affordable healthcare will require the genius of nursing. We have no choice. The public is depending on us, and the stakes are too high for us not to emerge as leaders in this public arena. It is time to engage our power, mobilize our vast numbers, and embrace our special relationship with the public in order to create a true transformation of healthcare. Drs. Grossman and Valiga have provided the nursing profession with a blueprint to help us assume this daunting responsibility.

Melanie C. Dreher, PhD, RN, FAAN
Dean and Professor
College of Nursing
University of Iowa
Iowa City, Iowa

Preface

The New Leadership Challenge: Creating the Future of Nursing has been written as a reference book and textbook for undergraduate or graduate students in nursing, as well as for nurses in practice. It provides an overview of major ideas related to the multidimensional concept of "leadership" and explores those ideas at various levels of one's career development: beginning, intermediate, and advanced. Each chapter includes learning objectives, a synthesis of extensive readings (from nursing, and more often, nonnursing literature) on the specific topic, and a variety of critical thinking exercises that are designed to help the reader better understand the topic and its relation to leadership and the development of individuals as leaders. Resources from the arts and humanities that relate to the specific top and that enhance learning about it are provided, and examples from clinical practice are included.

Unlike many other textbooks and resource books that address leadership, this book takes that charge seriously. In many other books, particularly those written by and for nurses and nursing students, the authors confuse leadership with management and end up focusing more on management than on leadership. Perhaps that is because the phenomenon of leadership is more elusive than that of management and because one cannot outline "steps" of leadership as one can do with management (e.g., planning, delegating, budgeting).

This book takes on the challenge of exploring the elements of true leadership, particularly in the "new world" context we face continually. It explores various definitions and conceptualizations of leadership, examines extant theories of leadership, analyzes the notion of vision and visionary leadership, and tackles the intricacies of leader-follower relationships. The importance of followership, the facilitation of change, the management of conflict, the use and abuse of power, gender issues in leadership, and the development of oneself and of others as leaders all are discussed. In essence, then, this book takes a broad look at the complex phenomenon of leadership for a new millennium and examines multiple dimensions of it.

The major points made throughout this book and its unifying elements are as follows: (1) although leadership and management are related, the are *not* one and the same; (2) leadership is not an innate ability but one that can be learned and developed through conscious and purposeful effort; (3) each of us can be and, perhaps, needs to be a leader if nursing is to advance as a profession and have a significant impact in the twenty-first century; and (4) there are ways in which each of us can develop as a leader throughout our careers. These points are made and the goals of the book achieved through a balance of theoretical exploration, the extensive use of real-world examples from clinical practice and education, self-assessment exercises, and the integration of creative learning activities.

The New Leadership Challenge: Creating the Future of Nursing focuses on nurses and nursing. It does not confuse leadership and management. It also explores the multifaceted concept of leadership in depth. As such, it is of value to several audiences.

Most undergraduate programs include a course in nursing leadership. A study conducted by one of the authors and another colleague revealed, however, that although many courses carried the title "Nursing Leadership," most actually dealt with management and delegation. In a world where experts recognize clearly that what really is needed for the future is true leadership, *The New Leadership Challenge: Creating the Future of Nursing* meets a need, particularly for those undergraduate programs that already have or will soon have a course that addresses true leadership.

Most graduate programs focus on the preparation of graduates for leadership roles in the profession, so a book that addresses just that is most appropriate. Students preparing as educators or nurse practitioners do not want to use a text that "advertises" leadership but that "delivers" management; if they wanted management, they would have pursued an MBA or a graduate degree in nursing administration. Instead, they want a text that helps them understand what leadership is and how it relates to the roles for which they are preparing. This book meets that need.

Finally, this book serves as a valuable resource for nurses in clinical practice, nurse educators, and nurse administrators who see the need to learn more about the phenomenon of leadership and how to develop those abilities in themselves and in others (e.g., fellow clinicians, students, one's staff). One's ongoing education in an ever-changing world cannot be limited to clinical, teaching, or administrative knowledge and skills alone. It also must address broader knowledge and skills—such as those related to leadership—that are integral to one's practice.

One of the most important features of this book is the exposure to and integration of the extensive writings about leadership done by experts in that field; thus, the literature base for this book is not limited to nursing. This is designed to broaden the readers' perspectives and expose them to a much wider range of resources that can be tapped for ongoing personal development.

The New Leadership Challenge: Creating the Future of Nursing, as the title implies, also presents a clear orientation to the future. Using the writings of Wheatley (*Leadership and the New Science,* 1992) as a basis, the entire book is "framed" in the context of the future—what organizations are expected to look like in the future, the skills that people associated with those organizations will need to survive and thrive, the need to plan for a blending of professional and personal commitments, and so on. The old-model, hierarchic organization that characterizes so many healthcare agencies is expected to "die" very quickly, and people in those organizations will need to be able to function and provide leadership in a totally new kind of environment. This book is designed to help professional nurses make this transition.

In addition to these important features, *The New Leadership Challenge: Creating the Future of Nursing* offers several other unique features. First, it is accompanied by an instructor's guide that offers numerous teaching approaches that might be used with undergraduate or graduate students and with nurses in practice. The Instructor's manual also includes an annotated reference list, which is intended to familiarize instructors with the vast array of literature that is available on leadership and concepts related to it. Finally, this book is accompanied by regular updates on the World Wide Web concerning new developments in leadership, conferences related to leadership, and current literature from a variety of fields that relate to leadership and its components. Overall, this book—conceptualized in its broadest sense—is designed to be interactive, stimulating, creative, challenging, and thought-provoking.

The intent of this book is to help nurses and nursing students explore the many facets of leadership and examine strategies that will aid them in (1) seeing themselves as potential leaders, (2) developing skills needed to function as leaders, and (3) taking on the challenges of a leadership role in the current and future healthcare setting. It challenges the reader's thinking, presents new ways to conceptualize leadership, and prepares nurses for their role as leaders in creating a preferred future for nursing. Readers are invited to open their minds to new perspectives; entertain the notion that the chaotic, uncertain world of today and tomorrow presents tremendous opportunities for nurse leaders to influence the future of our profession; and think of themselves as leaders who can develop in that role throughout their careers. We welcome you to the world of *The New Leadership Challenge: Creating the Future of Nursing.*

Contents

The New Leadership Challenge:

Creating the Future of Nursing

CHAPTER 1

The Nature of Leadership

Distinguishing Leadership from Management

The Nature of Leadership

Distinguishing Leadership from Management

Learning Objectives

- ☐ Compare and contrast the major theories of leadership.

- ☐ Discuss the essential elements of leadership.

- ☐ Describe the nine tasks of leadership.

- ☐ Distinguish leadership from management.

- ☐ Create a personal definition of leadership that reflects its essential elements.

INTRODUCTION

Chaos. Uncertainty. Unpredictability. Constant change. These are all characteristics of the world in which we now exist, and all expectations are that the world of the future will be even more chaotic, more uncertain, more unpredictable, and in even greater states of constant and unprecedented change and flux. Such worlds desperately call for new leaders. Indeed, "if there was ever a moment in history when a comprehensive strategic view of leadership was needed, ... this is certainly it" (Bennis & Nanus, 1985, p. 2).

Defining just what leadership is, who leaders are, what leaders do, and how leadership is different from management—a phenomenon with which it often is confused—is no easy task, however. This chapter is intended to address these questions and help the reader understand the complex, multidimensional concept we refer to as leadership. It also is intended to challenge readers to consider the leadership we need in nursing today, to think about themselves as leaders, and to reflect on how leadership responsibilities can be integrated into their roles as professional nurses.

For almost a century, writers have attempted to describe leadership and researchers have attempted to identify the defining characteristics of leaders. The outcome of all this study and analysis has been one very clear conclusion: "Leadership is one of the most observed and least understood phenomena on earth" (Burns, 1978, p. 2). It is multidimensional and multifaceted—a universal human phenomenon that many know when they see it, but few can clearly define.

In fact, "there are almost as many different definitions of leadership as there are persons who have attempted to define the concept" (Bass, 1990, p. 11). According to Bennis and Nanus (1985, p. 4):

Decades of academic analysis have given us more than 350 definitions of leadership. Literally thousands of empirical investigations of leaders have been conducted in the last seventy-five years alone, but no clear and unequivocal understanding exists as to what distinguishes leaders from non-leaders, and perhaps more important, what distinguishes *effective* leaders from *ineffective* leaders.

The lack of a "clear and unequivocal understanding" of leadership has led these experts on the subject to assert that "never have so many labored so long to say so little" (p. 4). Despite this situation, however, there is increasing clarity about what true leadership is and how it is different from a related phenomenon, that of management.

Theories of Leadership

GREAT MAN THEORY

Theories of leadership have evolved tremendously over the years (Bass, 1990, pp. 37–55). Among the earliest was the "Great Man Theory," which asserted that one was a leader if one was born into the "right" family—usually a family of nobility—and possessed unique characteristics, most of which were inherited. Although some individuals who were born into the "right" family did accomplish extraordinary things and did, in fact, change the course of history, the notion that "leaders are born, not made" did not capture the imagination of the masses, and it failed to recognize that there was more to leadership than having royal blood. Thus began the search for the traits or cluster of traits that would determine whether a person would be a leader.

TRAIT THEORIES

Personal trait theories of leadership attempted to distinguish leaders from other people and identify the universal characteristics of leadership. Not surprisingly, no qualities were found that were universal to all leaders, although a number of traits did seem to correlate with leadership (Bass, 1990): above average height and weight, an abundant reserve of energy, an ability to maintain a high level of activity, better education, superior judgment, decisiveness, a breadth of knowledge, a high degree of verbal facility, good interpersonal skills, self-confidence, and creativity. In addition to revealing no universal trait among leaders, these theories also failed to acknowledge the importance of the situation in which leadership occurred.

SITUATIONAL THEORIES

Situational theories, in comparison, gave clear recognition of the significance of the environment and the particular situation as factors in the effectiveness of a leader. They asserted that the leader was the individual who was in a position to institute change when a situation was ready for change. In other words, the leader did not plan for a change, nor was the leader chosen by a group of followers; he or she just "happened to be in the right place at the right time" and took the action that was needed to resolve a crisis or manage a problem. Although this view of leadership was broader than merely looking at one's heritage or specific traits, it still did not capture the complexity of the phenomenon and failed to acknowledge one very important element in a leadership "event"; namely, the followers.

MODERN THEORIES

More modern theories of leadership clearly recognize that effective leadership depends partly on the person of the leader, partly on the situation at hand, and partly on the qualities and maturity of the followers. In fact, most recent writings (Chaleff, 1995; Corona, 1986; DePree, 1992; DiRienzo, 1994; Kelley, 1992, 1993; Lee, 1993) assert that without followers, there is no leadership; therefore followers are a most significant element in the leadership "equation." Their needs, goals, abilities, sense of responsibility, degree of involvement, potentials, and so forth are all important in determining the effectiveness of a leader. In addition to acknowledging the significance of followers, more modern theories acknowledge that leadership is not a haphazard occurrence. Instead, it very much involves having a vision, communicating that vision to others, planning with followers on how to make the vision a reality, effecting change, managing conflict, empowering followers, serving as a symbol for the group, serving as a source of energy and renewal for the group, and taking responsibility for facilitating the ongoing development of followers.

Leadership is, indeed, a complex, multifaceted phenomenon that does not "just happen" and that is not limited only to an elite few. It can be learned. It is deliberative. It is not necessarily tied to a position of authority. And it is something that each one of us has the potential to do.

Leadership and Management

The vast array of textbooks on leadership—particularly textbooks in nursing—often are titled "leadership and management." A careful analysis of the content of those textbooks often reveals that a great deal of attention is given to management and very little to leadership. In fact, although the authors of many such textbooks make a point at the outset to claim that leadership and management are not the same thing, they often go on to use the terms interchangeably and imply that the only person who is providing leadership to a group is the person who is in the management position. Nothing can be further from the truth.

Although leadership and management are related phenomena and many managers are also leaders, they are not the same thing and should not be confused. Most important, one must remember that *leadership is not necessarily tied to a position of authority* and that each of us as a professional nurse has the potential, and perhaps the responsibility, to provide leadership—in our specific area of practice, our institutions, our professional organizations, our communities, and our profession as a whole.

TASKS OF LEADERSHIP

One of the most noted experts in the field of leadership, John Gardner, outlined nine tasks of leadership that help distinguish it from management. Those tasks of leadership (Gardner, 1989) are as follows:

1. *Envisioning goals:* pointing others in the right direction and helping the group deal with the tension between long- and short-term goals
2. *Affirming values:* regenerating and revitalizing the beliefs, values, purposes, and vision shared by members of the group, and challenging the values held by some
3. *Motivating:* unlocking or channeling motives that exist within members of the group, having and promoting positive attitudes, being creative, and encouraging others to be excited about the future and how they can be a part of it
4. *Managing:* planning, setting priorities, making decisions, facilitating change, and keeping the system functioning, all in an effort to move the group toward the goals and vision
5. *Achieving a workable unity:* establishing trust, striving toward cohesion and mutual tolerance, managing conflict, and "creating loyalty to the larger venture" (p. 29)
6. *Explaining:* helping others understand what the vision is, why they are being asked to do certain things, and how they relate to the larger picture
7. *Serving as a symbol:* serving as a risk taker and acting as the group's source of unity, voice of anger, collective identity, and continuity, as well as its source of hope
8. *Representing the group:* speaking and acting for or on behalf of the group and being an advocate for the group
9. *Renewing:* blending continuity and change and breaking routines, habits, fixed attitudes, perceptions, assumptions, and unwritten rules

Gardner (1989) asserts that the "*sine qua non* of leadership" (p. 29) is the ability to achieve a workable unity in the group and build community. He also notes that in the process of renewing, the leader must "keep a measure of diversity and dissent in the system [as

> *"The cautious seldom err."*
> —Confucius

a way to avoid] the trance of nonrenewal" (p. 33). In essence, "leadership is not tidy" (p. 33); it is more of an art than a science.

Management, in comparison, often is thought of as a science in which a series of steps can be followed to implement the role. Elements of the tasks of leadership will be explored in greater depth, but a careful look at how leadership differs from management may facilitate a more thorough understanding of leadership.

SPECIFIC DISTINCTIONS BETWEEN LEADERSHIP AND MANAGEMENT

Among those who have written extensively about the differences between leadership and management is Abraham Zaleznik (1981). Zaleznik asserts that leaders and managers are very different kinds of people: they differ in their motivation, in their personal history, and in how they think and act; they differ in their orientation toward goals, work, human relations, and themselves; and they differ in their worldviews.

> *"Managers are people who do things right. Leaders are people who do the right thing."*
>
> —Warren Bennis and
>   Burt Nanus

GOALS

Leaders are very active in formulating goals. They adopt a personal and active attitude toward those goals because they typically arise out of some personal passion for a better world and are mutually formulated. They shape ideas instead of merely responding to the ideas of others, and they act to change the way people think about what is desirable, possible, and necessary. Managers, by comparison, adopt impersonal attitudes toward goals because those goals often are formulated by someone farther up in the organizational hierarchy. Those goals are deeply embedded in the history and culture of the organization, and they arise out of necessity rather than passion and desire.

CONCEPTIONS OF WORK

Regarding their conceptions of work, leaders act to develop fresh approaches to long-standing problems and to open issues for new options. They are not satisfied with the status quo, and they tend to create an excitement in their work. Their instinct is to take risks, challenge "sacred cows," challenge existing assumptions, and ask "Why not?" For managers, work is seen as a task to be accomplished with the least amount of turmoil and the greatest amount of coordination and balance. They act to limit choices and "rock the boat" as little as possible. Their instinct, in contrast to leaders, is for survival.

RELATIONS WITH OTHERS

In their relations with others, leaders are very concerned with what events and decisions mean to those who are affected by them. They care about the people with whom they work, and they want to promote the development and individual creativity of their followers. They facilitate, focus on personal issues, and encourage the growth of others. Relationships with leaders may appear turbulent, intense, and at times, even disorganized because of the involvement of all concerned. Despite this ability to work effectively with others, leaders also are comfortable with solitary activity because it provides time for reflection, creative thinking, and incubation of ideas. Although managers often are thought of as "human engineers" (Holle & Blatchley, 1987) and they like working with people, they tend to maintain a lower level of emotional involvement in their relationships with employees. They assign, focus on personnel issues, and promote the growth of the organization. They prefer to reconcile differences, seek compromises, and not become involved with what events mean to others. Instead, managers are concerned with how events occur, how things get done, and whether tasks are accomplished, preferably in the most efficient, cost-effective manner.

SENSE OF SELF

Managers and leaders also have a different sense of self, according to Zaleznik (1981). Using the terms coined by William James many years ago, Zaleznik says leaders are "twice born" individuals—those who are separate from their environment, never "belong" to organizations, and have had many challenges in life. They are not threatened by the ideas of others because their sense of self comes from within, not from their roles or the expectations of others. Managers, on the other hand, often define themselves in terms of the organization and prefer not to have their ideas challenged. According to Zaleznik, they are "once born" individuals, whose lives are rather harmonious and who are very much influenced by others' opinions.

Table 1–1 summarizes these and other differences between leaders and managers. It is important to note that this table compares the extreme "ideal" leader with the extreme "ideal" manager for purposes of illustration. Although it may be difficult to do, many managers also serve as leaders in their organizations and people in positions of authority often are leaders; therefore the distinctions are not as clear-cut as Table 1–1 may suggest.

One point that is important to emphasize is that *one can be a leader without being in a position of authority*. It is this point that professional nurses need to keep in mind when they face the challenges of the practice arena: each one of us has the potential to provide leadership to create new futures, and we need not be in a hierarchical position of authority to do

Table 1-1 *Differences Between Leadership and Management*

	Leadership	**Management**
POSITION	Position is one selected or allowed by a group of followers.	Position is one appointed by someone higher in the organizational hierarchy.
POWER BASE	Power base comes from knowledge, credibility, and ability to motivate followers.	Power base is a legitimate one, arising from the position of authority.
GOALS/ VISIONS	Goals and visions arise from personal interests and passion and may not be synonymous with the goals of the organization.	Goals and visions are those espoused or prescribed by the organization.
INNOVATIVE IDEAS	Innovative ideas are developed, tested, and encouraged among all members of the group.	Innovative ideas are allowed provided they do not interfere with task accomplishment, but they are not necessarily encouraged.
RISK LEVEL	High risk, creativity, and innovation are involved.	Low risk, balance, and maintaining the status quo are involved.
DEGREE OF ORDER	Relative disorder seems to be generated.	Rationality and control prevail.
NATURE OF ACTIVITIES	Activities are those related to vision and judgment.	Activities are those related to efficiency and cost-effectiveness.
FOCUS	The focus is on people.	The focus is on systems and structure.
PERSPECTIVE	Long-range perspective, with an eye on the horizon, is critical.	Short-range perspective, with an eye on the bottom line, often dominates.
DEGREE OF "FREEDOM"	Freedom is freestanding and not limited to an organizational position of authority.	Freedom is tied to a designated position in an organization.
ACTIONS	Does the right thing (Bennis & Nanus, 1985, p. 21).	Does things right (Bennis & Nanus, 1985, p. 21).

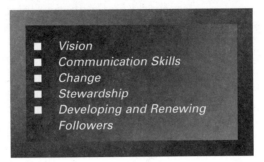

Box 1-1 *Elements of Leadership*

- Vision
- Communication Skills
- Change
- Stewardship
- Developing and Renewing Followers

that. In fact, if one considers how leaders "rock the boat," challenge existing ways of doing things, constantly ask "Why not?" questions, and are comfortable with turmoil—indeed, thrive on it—one can see that it sometimes is easier to be a leader if one is *not* in a hierarchical position of authority.

Elements of Leadership

As noted, leadership is a complex, multifaceted phenomenon that has been defined in hundreds of ways. Despite these myriad definitions, however, several elements of leadership recur in writings about the concept. Those elements—vision, communication skills, change, stewardship, and developing and renewing followers (see Box 1-1)—are discussed in depth to help the reader gain a better understanding of leadership.

VISION

One element of leadership about which few would argue is that of having, creating, and expressing a vision. Manfredi (1995) asserts that one of the primary roles of leaders is that of creating visions— "engag[ing] in the process of traveling into the future" (p. 62). Leadership involves dreaming of possibilities, believing that there can be a better world, exploring uncharted waters, and asking questions such as "Why not?"

> *"Leaders can conceive and articulate goals that lift people out of their petty preoccupations, carry them above the conflicts that tear a society apart, and unite them in a pursuit of objectives worthy of their best efforts."*
>
> —John Gardner

The significance of vision to leadership has been identified by numerous experts in the field (Bennis, 1989; DePree, 1989; Gardner, 1990; Kouses & Posner, 1987; Nanus, 1992; Phillips, 1997). In fact, the ability to see a new world or a different world and mobilize others to help make it a reality is one of the hallmarks of leadership. Consider the following examples of individuals and their dreams, many of which became realities as a result of the individual's determination, persistence, and passion:

> *"Cautious, careful people always casting about to preserve their reputation and social standing, never can bring about a reform. Those who are really in earnest must be willing to be anything or nothing in the world's estimation."*
>
> —Susan B. Anthony

- Henry Ford: affordable cars for "common" people
- Mother Teresa: compassionate care for the poorest of the poor
- Martin Luther King, Jr.: racial equality
- Candy Lightner: reduced drunk driving fatalities
- Mahatma Gandhi: freedom of the people of India
- Steve Jobs: desktop computers for personal use
- Robert Pittman: a "marriage" between rock music and television
- Fred Smith: overnight mail and package delivery, 365 days of the year
- Sam Walton: affordable shopping in a family-oriented store
- Florence Nightingale: reduced battlefield fatalities resulting from poor care

Although we think of these individuals today as major figures in our nation's or world's history, they were little-known men and women when their visions began to take shape, when they began talking to others about their vision, and when they initiated actions to turn those dreams into reality. As a result of the dreams and visions of men and women who, at the time of their initiation of ideas, were not well known at all, we now see most people owning cars, the worldwide impact of the Sisters of Charity, greater racial equality, the effectiveness of Mothers Against Drunk Driving (MADD), the positive outcomes of nonviolence, freedom of people in various parts of the world, the success of Wal-Mart and Federal Express, a computer in many homes and offices, the impact of Music Television (MTV) on our nation's youth, and more scientific and nursing-oriented approaches to healthcare.

As a professional nurse in practice, each of us has some vision of a better world. We might envision greater involvement of patients' families in care decisions or a more powerful role for the professional nurse on the healthcare team. We might see a more effective way to prepare patients to make the transition from the critical care unit to a step-down unit or from the hospital to home care. Or our vision may be for a longer hospital stay for mastectomy or other patients or greater autonomy for the nurse in making referrals to needed services.

Whatever the vision, if it is something about which we care, as leaders, we cannot sit idly by and wait for others to "make it happen." As leaders, we must talk about our vision to other nurses, our nurse managers and administrators, patients, patients' families, other health professionals, members of the media, legislators, in fact, anyone who will or who should listen. We must be passionate about the "little corner of the world" we think needs change and take every opportunity to do something to make that change happen. We do not have to be in positions of authority to raise the issues, to argue the necessity for the change, to elicit support for the idea, to speak eloquently and enthusiastically about possible solutions, or to convince others that it is a vision worth working toward. But what we *do* have to have is the vision.

> *"The secret of leadership is ... enthusiasm: winning others to your ideas by the joy you yourself feel in them."*
> —J. Donald Walters

COMMUNICATION SKILLS

As can be seen from the preceding discussion and from a review of Gardner's (1989) tasks of leadership, leadership involves communicating one's ideas and visions, explaining to others (e.g., followers, group members) how that vision has relevance for them and how they can be a part of making it a reality, and inspiring others to invest their energies on behalf of the group and the goal. In essence, excellent communication skills are essential for effective leadership.

Individuals who have great ideas but refuse to share them with others or who communicate them in a way that does not generate excitement in others are not likely to see their visions become reality. Individuals who cannot help others see clearly what the vision is probably will not be very effective in convincing those potential followers to "join in the struggle." And individuals who are unable to listen to the ideas of others, respond to their suggestions, and convey an enthusiasm for input from all group members are not likely to be able to facilitate change, sustain an effort over time, or effectively manage the conflict that is almost certain to arise as new goals are being realized.

One of the areas in which nurses are most skilled is communication. Nurses know how to listen. They know how to encourage people to keep trying when there seems to be no hope of success or when trying is extraordinarily difficult. They know how to encourage others to respond openly. And they know how to avoid barriers to communication. Therefore, nurses are particularly advantaged when one examines this element of leadership, and they should use this skill to its fullest.

The public puts a great deal of trust in nurses, and the credibility of nurses is strong in the eyes of patients, families, legislators, and the general public. Nurses who are providing leadership would therefore do well to take advantage of this trust and credibility by communicating their vision at every opportunity. Such opportunities are, in fact, more available than many nurses realize: serving on a committee at one's institution or in one's professional association, speaking at a conference, writing for a professional journal or a local newspaper or organizational newsletter, meeting with a legislator, talking with patients and their families, being interviewed on a campus radio station, holding office in one's professional association, campaigning for a candidate or a particular issue, confronting a healthcare team member, networking at professional meetings, forming alliances with other healthcare professionals, seeking and using a mentor, and so on. We are limited only by our own imagination and our own willingness to take risks.

CHANGE

If leadership involves articulating and realizing visions, the process by which that happens is the change process. Indeed, "learning to lead is, on one level, learning to manage change" (Bennis, 1989, p. 145). Leaders therefore need to be effective change agents, knowing when change is needed, "stretch[ing] the imagination of followers" (Manfredi, 1995, p. 63) to appreciate the need for change, planning effectively for change to occur, involving those who will be affected by change in the process, helping others realize their role in making change and creating new worlds, maintaining a positive attitude throughout the challenges of change, and knowing when to maintain the status quo.

As Gardner (1990, p. 124) noted, "leaders must understand the interweaving of continuity and change." They must realize that not all change is good or necessary and that changing only for the sake of changing is not always healthy. Therefore continuity often is what a group needs, at least for a certain period. But leadership also involves a willingness to create change and manage the chaos that often is associated with change. It involves being willing to risk failure rather than waiting for "guaranteed" success, and it involves keeping focused on the goal or vision.

Professional nurses have a responsibility to create change in their work or professional arenas. Nurses who are dissatisfied with the intake form used with new patients, for example, thinking it is not complete enough to provide an adequate database to plan long-term home care, can complain about the form to their colleagues and "blame" someone else for its inadequacies. But the professional nurse who is a leader will do more than just complain. That nurse will outline what is needed on an intake form to make it complete, perhaps test it out in practice (by informally adapting the existing form) to see how workable it

> *"Leadership is action, not position."*
> —Donald H. McGannon

is and whether it really provides the kind of data necessary to plan care, develop a plan for pilot testing of a revised form on a wider scale, and propose how the new form could be integrated into the admission standards for nurses in that agency. Such an approach creates change that is intended to improve the overall quality of patient care, and although it may take more effort than merely complaining about the inadequacies of the existing intake form, the outcomes seem worth the effort. Leaders do not need to be in positions of authority, and they do not need to wait for "guaranteed" success before trying new approaches and creating change.

STEWARDSHIP

"Stewardship is to hold something in trust for another" (Block, 1993, p. xx). It has to do with serving others, rather than serving our own self-interests or attempting to control others, and it involves a balance of power. In essence, stewardship incorporates "engendering partnerships" (Block, 1993, p. 6) and empowerment.

Block (1993) titles his first chapter "Replacing Leadership with Stewardship" and describes leadership as "inevitably associated with behaviors of control, direction, and knowing what is best for others" (p. 13), noting that it "does not leave much room for the concept of partnership" (p. 17). Based on the previous discussion, Block's definition may be an appropriate one for management, but it is not at all consistent with leadership the way it has been described here. Therefore leadership and stewardship are not necessarily opposites or incompatible phenomena. In fact, Block's discussion of stewardship as "creating something we care about so we can endure the sacrifice, risk, and adventure that commitment entails" (p. 10) is congruent with the elements of leadership described previously; namely, deep commitment, risk taking, high energy, working with others, and an enormous investment of self.

If leaders are to move forward with creating new worlds and helping visions become realities, they must have a sense of stewardship. They must feel responsible for the "larger picture," oversee the implementation of change, ensure that it is the overarching vision that drives decisions and actions, establish partnerships with followers or group members, and give their personal self-interests a "back seat."

Professional nurses at all levels need to have a sense of stewardship about their practice arenas—whether that be in the clinical area, education, administration, or research—and be concerned with overall excellence in those arenas. Educators, for example, who have a vision of creating positive learning experiences for students—where they are fully engaged in the learning process, work collaboratively with each other, are excited about what they are learning, use their creative and other potentials to the fullest, and use the teacher as a guide and a resource to facilitate their own learning—cannot be concerned with doing this only in their own courses. If they are to be leaders and demonstrate the essential element of stewardship, there must be an effort to see that such positive learning experiences are provided for students throughout the curriculum and a willingness to oversee that what is being done in the name of "positive learning experiences" is based on theory and research.

DEVELOPING AND RENEWING FOLLOWERS

Finally, leadership involves the continual development of followers and ongoing renewal of their commitment, understanding, and involvement. In fact, Tichy (1997) asserts that one of the truly defining characteristics of leaders is their investment in creating leaders all around them.

More than accomplishing tasks or meeting deadlines, "leadership is about taking people to places where they have never dared to go . . . and building into the future by developing the abilities of others" (Tichy, 1997, p. xiv). Leaders who have a vision for the future need to ensure that there are people to carry that vision forward and continue to work to make it become a reality. Building toward a vision requires collaboration between leaders and followers, as well as a cadre of effective followers who themselves provide leadership.

It is the leader's responsibility to build such a cadre and develop the next generation of leaders. Because "all people have untapped leadership potential" (Tichy, 1997, p. 6), part of the leader's role is to recognize that potential and capitalize on it so that an effort or change can be sustained. Developing and renewing others can occur through personal attention, role modeling, precepting, and mentoring, each of which are described briefly to point out their similarities and differences.

PERSONAL ATTENTION

Personal attention involves the personal guidance one gives to another. It requires that the strengths, limitations, and goals of the "recipients" are known and are used as a basis for the challenges presented to those individuals, the opportunities made available to them, and the expectations that are set regarding their contributions to the group.

ROLE MODELING

Role modeling occurs when a more experienced individual performs a role in such a way that novice leaders follow the experienced individual's actions, style, values, behaviors, and so on. Because one can be a role model for another without even knowing it, this method of developing and renewing others is considered a more passive approach.

PRECEPTING

Precepting is a strategy often used in nursing in which an experienced individual may be "assigned" to teach, guide, and assist another who is learning a role. Preceptors may be paid for their services, the preceptor relationship often has a specific time limitation, and specific responsibilities of the preceptor and preceptee are clearly outlined.

MENTORING

Mentoring, in comparison, is a purposeful relationship in which an experienced, accomplished individual chooses to enter into a relationship with a less experienced individual who shares certain values or goals, who is seen as having potential, whose "chemistry" matches that of the mentor, and who is willing to work with the mentor. Mentors "open doors" for protégés, give them critical feedback and personal guidance about career goals and other significant matters, and are willing to enter into a relationship that may last for many years. When true mentoring occurs, protégés may accomplish professional goals that far exceed those of the mentor.

It is clear that there are many approaches to developing and renewing followers. Some are conscious and purposeful (e.g., mentoring, personal attention), some are "assigned" (e.g., precepting), and some may occur without the leader even being aware of their occurrence (e.g., role modeling). Regardless of the strategy used, the leader is committed to the development of the followers and to their continued renewal and involvement.

CONCLUSION

Leadership is a complex, multifaceted phenomenon that is quite different from management. It is a talent that each of us has and that can be learned, developed, and nurtured. Most important, it is not necessarily tied to a position of authority in an organization.

Opportunities exist in all aspects of our lives for each of us to exercise leadership and to make a difference in the lives of others and in the directions of groups and organizations. Leaders do not need to be appointed or even "invited" to exercise leadership; they do it because they "care more than others think is wise; risk more than others think is safe; dream more than others think is practical; and expect more than others think is possible" (anonymous quote about attaining excellence).

"Never, never, never quit."
—Winston Churchill

Leadership is needed for growth and progress—of individuals, groups, organizations, and institutions. As Harry Truman once said, "In periods where there is no leadership, society stands still. Progress occurs when courageous, skillful leaders seize the opportunity to change things for the better." In this world of increasing chaos, uncertainty, unpredictability, holism, and constant change, leadership is desperately needed. Nowhere is this more evident than in today's healthcare arena.

Professional nurses are in an excellent position to provide leadership within their work settings, their professional associations, their communities, and society at large. Their skills of communication, their ability to work collaboratively with others, their sense of service to others, their well-established credibility, and their dreams for excellent patient care make them excellent candidates to provide this much-needed leadership.

Critical Thinking 1-1

Critical Thinking Exercises

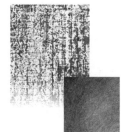

Given the opportunity to publish "the definitive definition of leadership," what would you write? How does your definition reflect the nine tasks of leadership and the essential elements of leadership?

Ask several nursing colleagues and several people outside the health professions (including children) to define leadership. What are the similarities in the definitions offered by these individuals? Are there any significant differences in their definitions? If so, what are they, and how do you explain those difference?

If an alien came to earth, approached you, and said, "I see you are a nurse. Take me to your leader," to whom would you take the alien? Who, in your opinion, is providing true leadership within the profession or even within your own institution? Why would you take the alien to this person?

Read *The Velveteen Rabbit* (Williams, 1975). What leadership concepts can you identify in this children's story? What can we learn about leadership from this story?

Read the poem "If" by Rudyard Kipling. How do you think this relates to leadership and to the art of becoming a leader?

"If"

by Rudyard Kipling

If you can keep your head when all about you
Are losing theirs and blaming it on you;
If you can trust yourself when all men doubt you
Yet make allowance for their doubting, too;
If you can wait and not be tired of waiting,
Or being lied about, don't deal in lies.
Or being hated, don't give way to hating,
And yet not look too good nor talk too wise;

If you can dream and not make dreams your master;
If you can think and not make thoughts your aim;
If you can meet with triumphs and disaster
And treat those two impostors just the same;
If you can bear to hear the truths you've spoken
Twisted by knaves to make a trap for fools,
Or see the things you gave your life to, broken
And stoop to build them up with worn-out tools;

If you can make one heap of all your winnings
And risk it on one turn of pitch and toss,
And lose and start again at your beginnings
And never breathe a word about your loss;
If you can force your heart and nerve and sinew
To serve your turn long after they are gone,
And so hold on when there's nothing in you
Except the will that says to them "hold on;"

If you can talk with crowds and keep your virtue,
Or walk with kings nor lose the common touch;
If neither foes nor loving friends can hurt you;
If all men count with you but none too much,
If you can fill the unforgiving minute
With sixty seconds worth of distance run—
Yours is the world and everything that's in it,
And—which is more—you'll be a man, my son!

References

Bass, B.M. (1990). *Bass and Stogdill's handbook of leadership* (3rd ed.). New York: Free Press.

Bennis, W. (1989). *On becoming a leader*. Reading, MA: Addison-Wesley.

Bennis, W., & Nanus, B. (1985). *Leaders: The strategies for taking charge.* New York: Harper & Row.

Block, P. (1993). *Stewardship: Choosing service over self-interest*. San Francisco: Berrett-Koehler.

Burns, J.M. (1978). *Leadership*. New York: Harper Torchbooks.

Chaleff, I. (1995). *The courageous follower: Standing up to and for our leaders*. San Francisco: Berrett-Koehler.

Corona, D.F. (1986). Followership: The indispensable corollary to leadership. In E.C. Hein & M.J. Nicholson (Eds.), *Contemporary leadership behavior: Selected readings* (3rd ed.) (pp. 87–91). Boston: Little, Brown.

DePree, M. (1989). *Leadership is an art*. New York: Dell.

DePree, M. (1992). *Leadership jazz*. New York: Doubleday Currency.

DiRienzo, S.M. (1994). A challenge to nursing: Promoting followers as well as leaders. *Holistic Nursing Practice 9*(1), 26–30.

Gardner, J.W. (1990). *On leadership*. New York: Free Press.

Gardner, J.W. (1989). The tasks of leadership. In W.E. Rosenbach & R.L. Taylor (Eds.), *Contemporary issues in leadership* (2nd ed.) (pp. 24–33). Boulder, CO: Westview Press.

Holle, M.L., & Blatchley, M.E. (1987). *Introduction to leadership and management in nursing* (2nd ed.). Boston: Jones & Bartlett.

Kelley, R. (1993). How followers weave a web of relationships. In W.E. Rosenbach & R.L. Taylor (Eds.), *Contemporary issues in leadership* (3rd ed.) (pp. 122–133). Boulder, CO: Westview Press.

Kelley, R. (1992). *The power of followership: How to create leaders people want to follow and followers who lead themselves*. New York: Doubleday Currency.

Kouses, J.M., & Posner, B. (1987). *The leadership challenge*. San Francisco: Jossey-Bass.

Lee, C. (1993). Followership: The essence of leadership. In W.E. Rosenbach & R.L. Taylor (Eds.), *Contemporary issues in leadership* (3rd ed.) (pp. 113–121). Boulder, CO: Westview Press.

Manfredi, C. (1995). The art of legendary leadership. *Nursing Leadership Forum 1*(2), 62–64.

Nanus, B. (1992). *Visionary leadership*. San Francisco: Jossey-Bass.

Phillips, D.T. (1997). *The founding fathers on leadership*. New York: Warner Books.

Tichy, N.M. (1997). *The leadership engine: How winning companies build leaders at every level*. New York: HarperBusiness.

Williams, M. (1975). *The velveteen rabbit*. New York: Avon Books.

Zaleznik, A. (1981). Managers and leaders: Are they different? *Journal of Nursing Administration 11*(7), 25–31.

CHAPTER 2

The New World and New Leadership

*Changing Our Thinking
about Leadership*

The New World and New Leadership

Changing Our Thinking about Leadership

Learning Objectives

☐ Define the new leadership that is necessary for nurses to adopt to participate successfully in and shape the healthcare system of today and tomorrow.

☐ Examine how chaos creates new opportunities for nurses to function as leaders in the healthcare delivery system.

☐ Describe how each of the following theories are congruent with the new leadership: quantum, developmental, cognitive, and perspective transformation.

☐ Identify how the new leadership influences the nursing profession, as well as individual nurses throughout their careers.

☐ Describe strategies to assist nurses' development as new leaders.

INTRODUCTION

Downsizing, re-engineering, merging, partnerships, acquisitions, and affiliations are what we hear about, read about, and talk about in the late 1990s. All organizations, particularly those in health-care, are experiencing one or more of these changes as evidenced by the 85 percent of nurse executives who, in reference to a national survey regarding the impact of organizational design on nursing, reported that their institution had already gone through or was in the process of redesign (Gelinas & Manthey, 1997).

To continue to participate successfully in healthcare, nursing will continue to need to find ways to use resources wisely, validate the effect of nursing interventions on patient outcomes, and develop new ways to provide quality and cost-effective care. Mechanisms by which these goals can be accomplished include focusing on health promotion in all types of care settings, encouraging multidiscipli-nary collaboration, integrating outcome assessment into our daily work as nurses, and "retooling" so that nurses can practice more autonomously and accountably as patient advocates.

To achieve such goals, however, all registered nurses (RNs) and advanced practice nurses (APNs) must think in a whole new way. Being confident and competent is consistent with the new view of leadership that nurses will need to have as they solidify their roles in the healthcare arena. Indeed, it is time to embrace the countless "problems" of organizational downsizing and look at each one of these problems as a challenging opportunity.

To implement change, a new way of leading healthcare reform must develop, and this "new way" is something quite different from management, as noted previously. We are now in a new age of healthcare (Porter-O'Grady, 1997). There are a plethora of articles and books discussing the use of unlicensed assistive personnel (UAPs), patient-focused organizational redesign (PFOR), managed care, capitation, the move from illness to health promotion, and team building, to name some of the issues. What is not reported, however, are outcome studies of the effects of these changes on care quality or specific ways in which healthcare providers, especially nurses, need to re-tool and think in new ways in order to remain significant players

"Do not follow where the path may lead. Go instead where there is no path and leave a trail."

—Anonymous

in this new age of healthcare (Porter-O'Grady, 1997). It is necessary to change our thinking so that nurses are able to engage in more independent decision-making, collaborate more effectively with nurse and nonnurse partners, and provide leadership.

Preparing Nurse Leaders

Sadly, many nurses are not prepared for the role they will need to assume in acute-care institutions, home care, or other settings, and they become overwhelmed all too quickly. This chapter is designed to help nurses change their minds about leadership and their roles as leaders so that they can more effectively participate in the new and ever-evolving healthcare field. In a study by Manfredi and Valiga (1990), a sample of baccalaureate programs were reviewed to evaluate whether the curricula focused more on the art of leadership or on the science of management. These authors found that most of the programs were teaching management. They also reported that faculty generally viewed "leadership" and "management" as synonymous.

In addition, nurses need to be better able to work in groups, especially with healthcare team members of other disciplines. Koerner (1997) interviewed two nursing leaders (K. Vestal and K. Ehrat) who are already thinking in a different way. Kathleen Vestal's advice to nurses is, "If you don't like change, get out of nursing . . . and if you want to stay in nursing, become part of the bigger world" (pp. 1–2). Karen Ehrat says, "There is a need for an integrated approach to education so nurses do not receive just a single discipline perspective" (p. 1). Ehrat reiterates that all disciplines bring strengths to the healthcare team; they cannot be allowed to compete with one another but must collaborate with and support each other. Perhaps a new way of thinking about leadership will assist nurses in appreciating themselves and seeing the value of their own, as well as their partners', contributions.

Developing Leadership

We are moving from the Scientific Age, with its emphasis on short- and long-term planning, predicting patient acuity, using formulas to provide staff coverage, and following bureaucratic procedures and policies, to getting tasks done, a New Science Age that stresses empowerment of all, creating while doing, evaluating processes and outcomes and collaborating as a team. Such a change requires us to exercise leadership in an entirely new way.

Covey (1996) describes three characteristics a leader must possess for a successful experience in growing and learning: vision, courage, and humility. Having a dream or vision is imperative, but one must have courage to continue to define it among a group and, at the same time, be humble enough to know when to redefine it to meet the needs of the changing times and to prepare for the future. Bennis and Nanus (1995) describe leadership as encompassing vision, the ability to communicate effectively, the ability to be steadfast, and the ability to demonstrate positive self-regard. Having the ability to consistently propel a vision in a group or organization takes self-confidence and assertiveness. Parse (1997) echoes Covey's and Bennis and Nanus's thoughts when she describes leaders as people who are committed to a vision, are willing to risk being challenged by others, and demonstrate a reverence for others.

For example, to change our nursing task orientation to a patient outcome focus, nurses can use leadership skills. If our vision was one of nurses working collaboratively with other healthcare members to provide care that best facilitates positive patient outcomes, the monitoring of clients for beneficial or untoward sequelae of nursing, medical, and pharmacological interventions would be done in collaboration with physicians and pharmacists, not in isolation. Practices that challenge the traditional "sacred cows" of the medical model of practice have to be adopted so that the vision of nurses providing nursing care and nursing being recognized as a means to obtaining positive patient outcomes is to be achieved.

Nursing leaders have been developing nursing diagnoses and a taxonomy of nursing interventions since the 1980s. Despite these efforts, however, we are still carrying out medical orders. What is needed is for nurses to define what nursing is and wants to be and then work as a unified body to achieve those goals. The current chaotic state of healthcare provides a window of opportunity for this vision to be realized. (See Chap. 7 for strategies leaders can use to take advantage of these opportunities.) We need to work to ensure a focus on excellence as well as on the bottom line. Nursing leaders must clearly identify responsibilities of RNs, APNs, and nonlicensed assistive personnel, and they must guide us in creating and strengthening new roles for nurses. With leaders who employ a new way of thinking about leadership, all of us can be successful in advancing our profession.

Chaos Faced by Nurses

As a new century dawns, nurses in practice must face the challenge of constant and multidimensional chaos. Nurses must have an extensive knowledge base, the abilities required to perform highly sophisticated technological skills, the decision-making and critical thinking skills that are essential to practice, and the capability of managing multiple problems simultaneously.

How does one have a vision, feel courageous, or feel humble when faced by these kinds of challenges and the kinds of problems being experienced by today's patients? To add to this chaos, it is possible that there is no experienced nurse with whom one can discuss problems, other staff members are overwhelmed by the amount and intensity of their own caseloads, the manager is not available, and resources are in short supply. Most nurses eventually get answers for their questions, and they may even get some help from their peers or a clinical resource person who is on call for the entire institution. When one regularly feels that he or she does not know enough, when advice or counsel is not readily available, when human and material resources are in short supply, and when effective leadership seems absent, however, the world seems chaotic and the individual is overwhelmed. The environments in which many nurses now practice are chaotic. But chaos is not all bad.

Chaos Theory

Vicenzi, White, and Begun (1997) suggest nurses take another look at their situations and view them as "complex, dynamic, and unpredictable" (p. 26) rather than hopeless. These authors acknowledge that nurses are in chaos, as is the whole healthcare system, but chaos theory implies that hidden within this seemingly total disorganization are patterns of order.

"*Chaos*" is a scientific term meaning "the apparently irregular, unpredictable behavior of deterministic, nonlinear systems" (Vicenzi, White, & Begun, 1997, p. 26). Wheatley (1992) says computers have awakened us to the true definition of chaos because of their ability to store megadata. Millions of pieces of data can be displayed at any one time on any screen. The system allows the millions of bytes of data to be displayed in what appears to be a chaotic mess, but as one tracks the computer screen, rapidly moving lines seem to appear and connect all of the pieces of data. Thus what appeared to be chaos actually takes an orderly shape that we may not have been able to visualize without a computer (p. 122).

Think about the last time you had an emergency patient situation—didn't everyone pitch in during the code? There were no formalities, and if the patient's situation further deteriorated, the code team probably became more collegial and informal as everyone tried harder. This is easily correlated to what happens in a bureaucratic organization when uncertainty increases. People tend to use more personal and group approaches (Kouzes & Posner, 1995, p. 86) as they come together for the common good, and this often occurs unconsciously. Leaders can be instrumental at times like this by using the chaos and the ultimate changes it produces as a positive opportunity. In other words, "growth is found in disequilibrium not in balance" (Wheatley, 1992, p. 20).

Challenging problems provide people with opportunities for great success. Sweating a bit or being a little anxious about something usually leaves us exhilarated after the problem has been resolved. The healthcare chaos that currently surrounds us is one such challenging problem. As a result, we may secure an even stronger role for nurses and identify more creative ways to provide high-quality and cost-effective care.

An example may help illustrate this point. Many in nursing bemoan the loss of the 80 percent professional staff and 20 percent nonprofessional staff mix we enjoyed in the 1980s and the reality of the current 60 percent professional staff and 40 percent nonprofessional staff mix in some hospitals today. However, until it can be documented that care is better and costs can be maintained with more professional staff, it is unlikely that the proportion of professional staff will increase. It would be contrary to the new science of leadership philosophy, however, to propose a quantitative study measuring cost-effectiveness. Instead, the new science perspective would encourage the emergence of creative leaders who are willing to stray from set formulas and achieve the right mix of staff for their individual units by experimenting until the best mix is found. For example, a proposal of gradually decreasing professional staff and increasing unlicensed personnel would be more tolerable than just eliminating RN positions. In addition, having an available RN "pool" would allow nurses to be called in when patient acuity justified professional care. The old bureaucratic way of thinking that a consistent number of staff members for every unit, with so many full-time equivalents (FTEs) of professional and nonprofessional staff, just does not work in a world characterized by chaos.

The new science philosophy recommends less prediction, prejudgment, and compartmentalization. Wheatley (1992) and Porter-O'Grady and Wilson (1995) suggest that we stop dwelling on tasks and instead focus on facilitating the processes needed to obtain desired goals. For example, nurse managers need to try new staffing patterns that acknowledge that a 60 percent professional and 40 percent nonprofessional staff mix (or an 80 percent professional and 20 percent nonprofessional or a 30 percent professional and 70 percent nonprofessional staff mix) is not ideal for every unit, but any number of patterns could work if staff learn to work with each other in new ways. Leaders need to concentrate first on the people who are working to achieve the goals and establishing positive relationships between and among them. Any number of tasks can then be accomplished. If people have a positive working relationship with each other, they are more likely to respect each other and more likely to achieve great things. As Wheatley says, "what gives power its charge, positive or negative, is the quality of the relationships" (1992, p. 39).

Some organizations are calling on nurses to navigate their institutions through this chaotic time, and nursing leaders are using a number of creative strategies to influence change, survive, and even grow. One of these strategies is "change magic" (Hernandez, Spivak, & Zwingman-Bagley, 1997, p. 38), the use of imagination in combining change theory with the knowledge of the customer, the art of nursing, and the attributes derived from chaos. Skills such as creativity, patient centeredness, coordination, multiple priority management, problem solving, critical thinking, and system navigation are identified as being necessary for nurses to use throughout their careers. Numerous theories support a new holistic view of leadership and find growth in chaos: quantum theory and the new science, developmental theory, cognitive theory, and perspective transformation.

Quantum Theory and the New Science

Wheatley (1992) was among the first to relate the changes we have witnessed in science to the need for a new view of leadership. She noted that "if we are to draw from the sciences to create and manage organizations, to design research, and to formulate hypotheses about organizational design, planning, economics, human nature, and change processes, then we need to at least ground our work in the science of our times" (p. 6). By "the science of our times," Wheatley is referring to new research in the disciplines of physics, biology, and chemistry, as well as to the theories of chaos and evolution, which span several disciplines. This new science focuses on relationships and a nonlinear approach, where the real and the potentially real are visualized simultaneously. It is a method of thinking that replaces our standard, orderly, goal-oriented perspective with a free-flowing, open-space, always-moving, anything-can-happen philosophy.

Wheatley (1992) recommends that we approach leadership through the lens provided by the new science and naturally occurring events. For example, after a storm, meteorologists can review storm patterns on a computer and visualize a pattern in what initially appeared to be chaos. Or we can reflect on the fact that a stream, which initially seems to be little more than a random collection of water, sand, rocks, and silt, actually is not random at all but is a carefully designed system in which all parts work together to allow flexibility and the capacity for change as the natural elements of storms, animals, and humans affect its path.

The new science says that living systems organize themselves by seeking order, but this order is not linear and predictive. Organizations, says Wheatley (1992), operate in the same way. They seek order, but not in a linear, hierarchical way. Thus leadership in an organization may best be provided by a social system comprising many leaders, not only one. Those who relate through coercion or with a disregard for others create negative energy, whereas those who are open to others and who see others in their fullness create positive energy. Perhaps by focusing on one non-professional staff member at a time and allowing a "connectedness" to occur between that individual and the other staff, a we-versus-they situation can be avoided. If each staff member can be empowered to visualize his or her own potential as well as that of each other, a more positive outlook regarding workload and quality of patient care will prevail.

Quantum theory suggests that an interface among all members of a group is critical. Each person needs to be acknowledged for his or her talents and potential, and each needs to be helped to grow. Perhaps we need to visualize the workforce as germinating seeds in space rather than on earth where gravity pulls the roots toward it and the stem grows away from gravity. In space, seeds grow every which way, not only upward from the ground, because there is no gravity to direct them. Likewise, people are not fixed entities gravitating toward one and only one spot and able to be predicted by a set of rules and expectations.

People need to be given the opportunity to grow in all kinds of ways—ways that are unknown to anyone until they happen. It is the task of the leader to encourage and facilitate such growth. Perhaps visualizing an organization as composed of Gumby-like figures that stretch and overlap with each other in more of a three-dimensional rather than linear structure would allow for greater diversity and uniqueness and open more avenues for communication. Work productivity cannot be predicted based on a given number of FTEs, certain types of patient hours, and acuity levels. Such task-oriented thinking is not what patient care is all about. Instead, our mindsets need to be more multidimensional and open to new possibilities and things that no one has thought of yet. Leaders are the key to success because they facilitate relationships, encourage growth, enjoy uncertainty, and are willing to take risks.

This new way of thinking about leadership in a global and limitless fashion, and realizing that each individual has a contribution to make is necessary if nursing is to succeed in delivering the highest-quality care. Valuing hard work and respecting one another are values that need resurrection and that must be pervasive. In other words, the whole culture of our practice settings needs reawakening. A job cannot be viewed as just a job but as a piece of an ever-changing plan that affects the greater goal of an organization. Each and every person must be respected as crucial to the greater goal. Biases, prejudices, insecurities, and preconceived judgments need to be worked out or left behind. When such an atmosphere exists, communication, mentoring, and collaboration are more likely to occur, and self-empowerment and group empowerment dominate. The change from a task-focused setting to more of a process-focused one allows followers and leaders to propel organizations and the individuals within them forward.

The world is moving out of the Industrial or Newtonian Age in which things were described in a linear way and we became accustomed to separating every system into parts, rather than dealing with the whole. Indeed, leaders are needed as the world moves toward a greater concern for wholeness, complexity, and interaction.

"We cannot assume we can see endings simply by defining what we want them to be" (Porter-O'Grady, 1997, p. 15). We have to use our imaginations and be more in tune with the idea that there is more to our work than assessing, planning, implementing, and evaluating. Nurses can no longer have tunnel vision and be task-oriented. Our whole philosophy of caring for the patient will have to be broadened, and for most of us, our whole way of living from task to task will have to change. Most RNs, the average of whom is 42.3 years old and has worked most of her or his 20-plus years (Brewer, 1997) in a very rigid organizational structure carrying out another profession's orders, will have to reorient themselves to nursing and leading with this new science of leadership perspective. The quantum mechanics framework of attending to naturally occurring events appreciates individuals for their knowledge and recognizes that they need tools and support, not direction and control (Porter-O'Grady, 1997).

Supporting Perspectives

The idea that people and organizations grow and evolve in response to challenges, disequilibrium, and change is not new, nor is it restricted to quantum mechanics or new science thinking. In fact, it is an idea that has been addressed by psychologists, educators, and nurse theorists. Examples of these follow.

Cognitive and intellectual development occur as one is increasingly able to use complex cognitive skills to analyze issues, manage changing circumstances, integrate multiple points of view, and make sound decisions independently (Perry, 1970). Individuals progress through stages of cognitive development, from seeing knowledge as finite and themselves as absorbers or memorizers of it, to viewing knowledge as relative and themselves as critical thinkers and lifelong learners (Valiga, 1983). Such changes in worldview, similar to any type of growth, occur as a result of disequilibrium (Valiga, 1983). When one's usual way of thinking is found to be lacking, one experiences disequilibrium and is challenged to think in new ways, ask new questions, and develop new strategies. The chaos and disequilibrium with which nurses in practice are challenged, therefore, can be viewed as a stimulus for growth and development. Nurses need to change their thinking about their role in healthcare, the kind of leadership needed in this arena, and their own responsibility to provide such leadership.

Erikson, a developmental theorist, stated that physical, emotional, and social factors have an effect on an individual's development (Erikson, 1963). He asserts that development is a mixture of maturation (the potential growth a person has inherited) and learning (knowledge to be gained). Behavioral theory says "there are no autonomous people since people are what they do and what they are reinforced for doing by conditions in their environment" (p. 36). Again, most nurses are working in the rigidly structured healthcare system and, without leadership ability, may not move out of adolescence or young adulthood stages. The nurse may be in the first stage of adulthood, the task of which is to master involvement with others occupationally. Mastery results in intimacy and solidarity, whereas failure results in isolation. The new leadership is based on relationships; therefore it is paramount that individuals accomplish this task so that they can be participating healthcare team members. The accomplishment of the generativity task for those aged 30 to 60 years leads to productive and creative work. For nurses to experience this generativity, they also need to have acquired leadership skills. Just as our lives can be viewed developmentally, so too can our organizational systems.

Only organizational structures that continue to be flexible and change (e.g., move up and down the developmental continuum) will be able to support the development of people in the organization. Sometimes, it is only when a person is pushed, such as when in a chaotic job setting or in severe conflict with one's peers to accomplish a task or tasks, does the individual actually develop and grow. Hence, developmental theory also is a proponent of disequilibrium not being a negative thing but rather a positive experience to enhance growth.

Fawcett (1995) explains that "each nurse, as well as the health care system itself, requires time to evolve from the use of individual, implicit frames of reference for nursing practice to an explicit model" (p. 532). The process that occurs during this period of growth when an individual has not clearly defined a frame of reference for nursing practice to a clearly defined conceptual model is perspective transformation. It is a developmental type of experience that depends on the kinds of experiences one has been exposed to in school or in the work setting. Using Fawcett's (1995, pp. 533–534) explanation of perspective transformation, one can visualize how leaders can assist nurses to identify their own ability to lead and hence grow in these chaotic times.

Stage 1, stability, reflects what many nurses are currently experiencing in their workplace. Nurses easily maintain the status quo because many were never encouraged to think of themselves as leaders. They accept the conditions of employment and often feel appreciative that they have jobs.

Stage 2, dissonance, moves one toward the revelation that all nurses can be leaders. It generally means the beginning of a reawakening to one's situation. Nurses who are experiencing dissonance are aware of the very chaotic times they are in and know they need to start to do something about this. They may share their feelings with peers and start speaking out when serious staffing problems or unsafe situations occur.

Stage 3, confusion, is when individuals gain courage from others who validate what they are feeling, speak openly about things not being right, and decide not to "put up with it anymore!"

Stage 4, dwelling with uncertainty, is when individuals speak out, but they do so sporadically because they may believe that they do not have the ability or strength to change things. ~~scattered~~

Stage 5, saturation, occurs when people feel confident they have collected the right information and spoken to the right people about a new way of doing things or delivering care.

Stage 6, synthesis, heralds the organization of data to formulate a plan to change an unacceptable situation. A plan is put into place because individuals cared enough to make a change.

Stage 7, resolution, indicates that the problems are beginning to be solved with the changes that were put into place.

In *stage 8, reconceptualization,* those who initiated the change continue to "work out some of the kinks" in the system and empower each other to continue to support and pursue the new way of doing things.

Stage 9, return to stability, indicates that the new change or way of doing things has now become a part of the milieu and is no longer being evaluated and scrutinized.

This framework can be another basis for arguing why we need to rethink about leadership because it depicts a change from nurses practicing in their own individual private way to an entire nursing staff using a shared model of practice. This is a good example of how something positive can come from living or working in chaos. Perspective transformation is a helpful process to use in assisting nurses to practice more autonomously. It also could assist in nursing in receiving a more equivalent piece of the healthcare dollar because it should assist in measuring tangible client outcomes, which are a direct result of nursing care.

CONCLUSION

We need to change our thinking about what leadership is to survive the tumultuous changes in healthcare. Chaos theory will assist us in understanding how the disorder and confusion we are feeling in our work settings today are equivalent to what happens in nature. The fact that the natural world we live in can automatically order itself after such turmoil is incredible. We have to realize that adapting the new science of leadership with its focus on empowering followers and alleviating the bureaucratic organizational structure will assist us in developing new ideas and new ways of working.

The transformation to managed care that so many nurses are currently confronting is certainly disheveling and chaotic, but it is necessary to change the hierarchical medical model on which the U.S. healthcare system has been based. This major paradigm shift should not only reduce costs but also improve the quality of healthcare. Quantum theory, cognitive theory, developmental theory, and perspective transformation frameworks provide further evidence that chaos and disequilibrium can be a positive instigators for growth and improvement. This new way of thinking about leading will help us provide a more collaborative and holistic approach to practice.

Critical Thinking Exercises

Explain how the new way of thinking about leadership described in this chapter can affect the way we conceptualize the role of the nurse today. How could you assist others in adapting this perspective?

_____

_____

Think about the environment in which you practice. Would you describe it as chaotic? If so, why? What contributes to the chaos? What have been the negative ways that you and others have dealt with this chaos? What positive strategies have been used? What patterns do you see in the midst of all this chaos?

_____

_____

Listen to a jazz musical selection with an extended "improv" (improvisational) piece. Despite the seemingly chaotic notes and chords, do you hear or feel any patterns or synchrony? How did you identify such patterns? (Note: This same exercise could be done by viewing a late Picasso painting or even watching a hockey game.)

_____

_____

Who do you think of as leaders where you practice? What characteristics of the new science of leadership do these people portray?

_____

_____

References

Bennis, W., & Nanus, B. (1995). *Leadership: The strategies for taking charge.* New York: Harper & Row.

Brewer, C. (1997). Through the looking glass: The labor market for RNs in the 21st century. *Nursing and Health Care Perspectives 18*(5), 260–269.

Covey, S. (1996). Three roles of the leader in the new paradigm. In F. Hesselbein, M. Goldsmith, & R. Beckhard (Eds.), *The leader of the future* (pp. 149–160). San Francisco: Jossey-Bass.

Erikson, E. (1963). *Childhood and society* (2nd ed.). New York: W. W. Norton & Co.

Fawcett, J. (1995). *Analysis and evaluation of conceptual models of nursing* (3rd ed.) (pp. 533–534). Philadelphia: F.A. Davis.

Gelinas, L., & Manthey, M. (1997). The impact of organizational redesign on nurse executive leadership. *Journal of Nursing Administration 27*(10), 35–42.

Hernandez, D., Spivak, L., & Zwingman-Bagley, C. (1997). Nurse leaders: Roles driving organizational transition. *Nursing Administration Quarterly 22*(1), 38–46.

Koerner, J. (1997). Profiles of leadership: A dialogue with two nurse revolutionaries. *Nursing Administration Quarterly 22*(1), 1–7.

Kouzes, J., & Posner, B. (1995). *The leadership challenge: How to keep getting extraordinary things done in organizations* (2nd ed.). San Francisco: Jossey-Bass.

Manfredi, C., & Valiga, T. (1990). How are we preparing nurse leaders? A study of baccalaureate curriculum. *Journal of Nursing Education 29*(1), 4–9.

Parse, R. (1997). Leadership: The essentials. *Nursing Science Quarterly 10*(3), 109.

Perry, W. (1970). *Forms of intellectual and ethical development in the college years: A scheme.* New York: Holt, Rinehart, & Winston.

Porter-O'Grady, T. (1997). Quantum mechanics and the future of healthcare leadership. *Journal of Nursing Administration 27*(1), 15–20.

Porter-O'Grady, T., & Wilson, C. (1995). *The leadership revolution in health care.* Gaithersburg, MD: Aspen Publishers.

Valiga, T. (1983). Cognitive development: A critical component of baccalaureate nursing education. *Image: The Journal of Nursing Scholarship 15*(4), 115–119.

Vicenzi, A., White, K., & Begun, J. (1997). Chaos in nursing: Make it work for you. *American Journal of Nursing 97*(10), 26–32.

Wheatley, M. (1992). *Leadership and the new science: Learning about organization from an orderly universe.* San Francisco: Berrett-Koehler.

CHAPTER 3

Followership and Empowerment

Followership and Empowerment

Learning Objectives

- ☐ Analyze the concept of followership.

- ☐ Examine elements of the follower role that are appealing and those that are not.

- ☐ Examine the similarities between leaders and followers.

- ☐ Articulate the interdependence between leaders and followers.

- ☐ Formulate strategies to develop oneself as an effective follower.

INTRODUCTION

In today's socio-technical organizations, the culture is collective (team), the expectation is involvement and investment, and the style of implementation is facilitative and integrative (Porter-O'Grady, 1993, p.•••.

In today's flatter, leaner environment, organizations and leaders cannot succeed without committed, contributing followers (Kelley, 1992, p. 200).

With the kind of organizational environments described above, it is clear that leaders will need to work collaboratively with followers if the organization is to succeed. Indeed, "any organization is a triad consisting of leaders and followers joined in a common purpose . . . Followers and leaders orbit around the purpose; followers do not orbit around the leader" (Chaleff, 1995, p. 11) (Fig. 3–1). Despite this need for collaboration, however, we know very little about followers and followership even though we are coming to know more and more about leaders and leadership.

Leadership and followership are two separate concepts, two separate roles that are complementary or reciprocal, not competitive. They are synergistic, "a dialectic . . . depend[ing] on each other for existence and meaning" (Kelley, 1992, p. 45). In other words, just as "up" has little meaning were it not for "down," the word "leader" has little meaning without the word "follower," and vice versa. In fact, *there can be no leaders without followers, and there can be no followers without leaders.*

No one person can know the best strategy, have the clearest vision, or identify the most effective approaches to solve problems. Instead, "all participants [need to be] recognized as full partners in the organizational venture . . . [and they need to be] co-leaders in the enterprise" (Sullivan, 1998, p. 469). Organizations of today and the next century need "a new, more democratic vision [that] . . . creates dynamic partnerships, combining the best of what we are collectively while empowering us as individuals" (Dreher, 1996, p. xiii). In other works, both leaders and followers are increasingly important (Fig. 3–2).

> *"The secret of leadership is ... the ability to inspire others with faith in their own high potential."*
> —J. Donald Walters

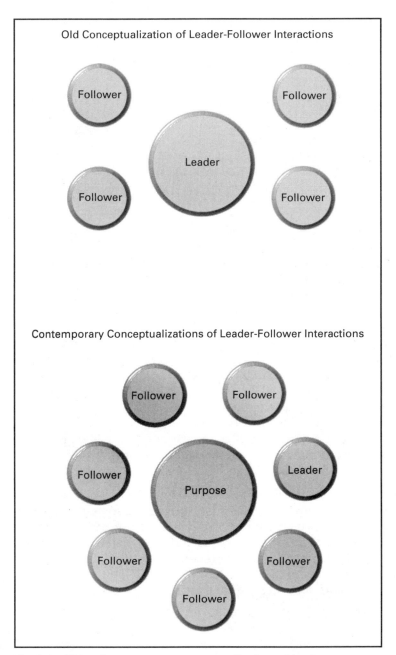

Fig. 3–1 *Old and contemporary conceptualizations of leader-follower interactions.*

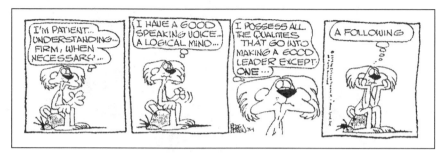

Fig. 3–2 *Leaders need followers.*

As many have noted, *leaders can be leaders only if they have followers.* Indeed, "to be a leader means generating followership" (Staub, 1996, p. 74) and "followership is the basis for all leadership" (Staub, 1996, p. 76). One author (Lundy, 1993, p. 21) flatly stated that "the ultimate criterion [in defining] a leader . . . is anyone who has followers." Despite these assertions, however, the concept of followership rarely is addressed to the same extent as the concept of leadership. There are no conferences held about followership; individuals do not seek consultation on how to be an effective follower; there is little, if any, content in educational programs on effective followership; and little has been written on the concept. Why does such a significant role receive so little attention? Does our emphasis on leadership "compensate for something in our culture or our organizations that fills us with an exaggerated need to promote leadership and to silence whatever haunts us about the notion of followership?" (Berg, 1998, p. 28).

Few would argue that followership is a neglected topic. In fact, a recent review of textbooks on nursing leadership and management (Anderson, 1999; Rocchiccioli & Tilbury, 1998; Swansburg & Swansburg, 1999; Yoder-Wise, 1999) revealed virtually no mention of the concept. And in a recent book titled *Strategies for the Future of Nursing* (O'Neil & Coffman, 1998), little mention is made of leadership and none of followership.

In one nursing leadership and management book, the word "follower" was used only as an example of a role someone in a group often takes to build and maintain the group; the follower was defined as "a group member who accepts the other group members' ideas and listens to their discussion and decisions" (Swansburg & Swansburg, 1999, p. 402). In this same book, the authors did talk about the mutual influence of leaders and those whom they lead; however, the authors chose to use the word "constituent" instead of "follower." Although they did not provide the reader with a reason for the choice of words, one might assume it has something to do with the negative connotations the word "follower" often carries.

In her review of her own path to leadership as the president of the American Nurses' Association, Joel (1999) said she was an "extraordinary follower . . . [who] learned the rules well and followed them exactly . . . [was] too intimidated to question authority . . . [and who] lacked confidence" (p. 17). She was, in essence, invisible.

One might conclude from these brief examples that there is something about the word "follower" or the notion of followership that is negative, demeaning, and unattractive. In reality, however, the follower role is a powerful one because "the responsibility for making the leader-follower relationship work remains with the 'follower'" (Berg, 1998, p. 33).

The Concept of Followership

Being a "good" follower takes special talents, just as being a "good" leader does. Conscious attention must be given to the development of followers and followership must be cultivated, just as leadership development and the cultivation of leadership are important. If we fail to remember that followership is voluntary, fail to convey the importance of followership, and fail to cultivate effective followers, leaders will be left without the support needed to realize visions, make change, and create a preferred future. In essence, when the cry goes out to "follow the leader," few will know who to follow or how to follow and little will be accomplished. Worse yet, the masses will not be prepared to identify the worthy leader and may follow the person with the loudest voice or the most charisma, as was the case with the Hitler Youth, the Jim Jones Guyana community, and the Waco, Texas, commune.

Followership is an art—a skill that can be learned, cultivated, and consciously developed and exercised. Followers need to be "self-directing, actively participating, practicing experts [who work] on behalf of the organization and the mutually agreed upon vision and goals" (Sullivan, 1998, p. 469). They need to trust others and be trustworthy themselves. They need to see themselves as a community,

> *"The final test of a leader is that he leaves behind him in other men the conviction and the will to carry on."*
> —Walter Lippman

think and act as a team, and invest energy in team building by focusing on the common goal and drawing on the strengths and talents of each member of the team. Followers need to know their own strengths and what their unique contributions to the effort can be; then they must complement each other's and the leader's specialties, strengths, and areas of expertise. They need to seek information so that they have the "larger picture," which allows them to participate fully and provide significant feedback. Followers should not invest their energy merely in their own or others' individual or personal agendas. They also should not ally themselves with group members whose goals are out of alignment with those of the rest of the team. They need to be counted on to "provide input that focuses on finding solutions, not just on articulating problems" (Sullivan, 1998, p. 478). They are expected to support the leader by asking questions, giving thoughtful feedback, working to achieve group goals, and providing encouragement when the leader takes a risk on behalf of the group (Corona, 1986); leaders, in return, are expected to support the followers by seeking their input, using their talents fully, and encouraging them to grow continually. Leaders and followers must "fuse to move together toward a common goal" (Joel, 1999, p. 30).

Followership also involves knowing when and how to assume the role of leader when necessary. "The organization is essentially a community of many leaders and many followers, frequently changing places depending on the particular activity that is occurring" (Sullivan, 1998, p. 477). "We all have the capacity to become either leaders or followers and both are necessary. There are no leaders without followers, and no matter how high you climb the leadership ladder, there is always the requirement to follow some of the time . . . These roles are not in competition, but rather natural compliments [sic] to one another's success" (Joel, 1999, p. 29).

A follower is an individual who takes another as a role model and who acts in accordance with, who imitates, and who supports and advocates the ideas and opinions of another (Brown, 1980). Without both leaders and followers, "there can be no unity, no successful goal-directed activity, and no true . . . achievement" (Brown, 1980, p. 357). But "taking another as a role model," "imitating," and "acting in accordance with another" do not mean that followers are passive, unthinking individuals who have no ideas of their own. On the contrary, "supporting and advocating the ideas and opinions of another" demands that the follower think critically about those ideas and opinions, have the skills to advocate for those ideas, and take an active role in providing support to the leader as the ideas are fully developed and advanced.

> *"The secret of leadership is ... never to ask of others what you would not willingly do yourself."*
>
> —J. Donald Walters

Types of Followers

Despite the vital role that followers actually play in effecting change and realizing visions, many still see the role as passive, dependent, unthinking, and lacking in status. Such negative perceptions of followers and followership are common, but they suggest that there is only one type of follower. Kelley (1992, 1998), on the other hand, suggests that there are several types of followers (Fig. 3–3), ranging from those who are vital to the success of the group or organization to those who are passive and unthinking:

- *Effective or exemplary followers:* These are the individuals who can function independently, who think critically about ideas that are proposed or directions that are suggested and who are actively involved. They will challenge the ideas of the leader, suggest alternative courses of action, and invest time and energy to arrive at the best possible solution for the group.
- *Alienated followers:* These are the individuals who are thinking critically about what the leader or other members of the group are suggesting, but they remain passive and perhaps even somewhat hostile. They may complain about "the way things are being done," are unhappy, and seem disengaged at times. Alienated followers will rarely invest time or energy to suggest alternative solutions or other approaches.
- *Yes people:* These are the conformists who are actively involved in the work of the group and who enthusiastically support the leader. They are eager to take orders, defer to the leader, yield to the leader's views and opinions, and please the leader, and they enjoy a great deal of structure, order, and predictability. "Yes" people are uncomfortable with having to make and live with decisions, and they find freedom almost terrifying. They do not initiate ideas, think for themselves, raise questions, critique the ideas of others, or challenge the group.
- *Sheep:* These are the passive individuals who are dependent and uncritical, going along with whatever the leader tells them to do. They are easily led and manipulated, lack initiative, require a great deal of direction, and never go beyond their given assignment. "Sheep" are not particularly committed to the goals of the group and do not invest themselves to any great extent to see that the group continues to move forward.

Types of followers, or followership styles, also have been described by Pittman, Rosenbach, and Potter (1998). Rather than using Kelley's (1992, 1998) "passive/active" and "independent/dependent" parameters, these authors use the dimensions

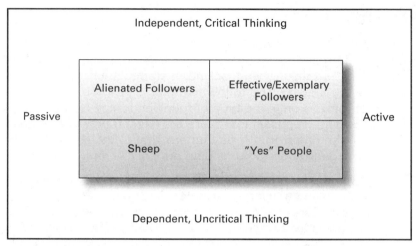

Fig. 3–3 *Types of followers. (Adapted from Kelley, R.E. [1998]. In praise of followers. In W.E. Rosenbach & R.L. Taylor [Eds.], Contemporary issues in leadership [4th ed.] [p. 98]. Boulder, CO: Westview Press; and Kelley, R. [1992]. The power of followership: How to create leaders people want to follow and followers who lead themselves [p. 97]. New York: Doubleday Currency.)*

of "performance initiative" and "relationship initiative" to define four followership styles (Fig. 3–4).

Performance initiatives relate to the follower's performance—how his assigned job gets done, how good the person is at what he or she does, the standards the person sets for himself or herself, how well the person works with others, and how valuable the person is to the organization. Relationship initiatives concern the follower's relationship to the leader—how much the person understands the leader's perspective, the person's willingness to give negative feedback or disagree with the leader, and how the person demonstrates his or her reliability and trustworthiness. Each of the four followership styles reflects extensive or limited activity in these dimensions:

- *Partner:* This follower is committed to high performance and to building a positive, reciprocal relationship with the leader. The partner may be thought of as a "leader-in-waiting" (Pittman, Rosenbach & Potter, 1998, p. 118).
- *Contributor:* This person does the job very well, is effective with coworkers, embraces change, and successfully balances work and other aspects of life. The contributor does not, however, try to understand the leader's perspective or promote the leader's vision, nor does he or she negotiate differ-

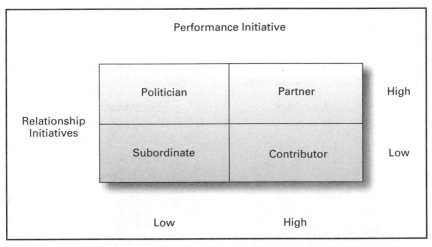

Fig. 3–4 *Followership styles. (Source: Pittman, T.S., Rosenbach, W.E., & Potter, E.H., III. [1998]. Followers as partners: Taking the initiative for action. In W.E. Rosenbach & R.L. Taylor [Eds.], Contemporary issues in leadership [4th ed.] [p. 113]. Boulder, CO: Westview Press.)*

ences maturely or communicate courageously (Chaleff, 1995; Pittman, Rosenbach, & Potter, 1998).

- *Politician:* This individual is highly sensitive to and skilled with interpersonal relationships. The person is willing to give honest feedback and supports the leader; however, he or she may neglect the job and have poor performance levels.
- *Subordinate:* This type of follower may be competent at assigned tasks and do what he or she is told, but there is no commitment to excellence in his or her performance. In addition, the subordinate is not particularly sensitive to relationships and does not make an effort to support the leader.

What nursing needs as we enter the new millennium are effective or exemplary followers or partners. Blindly following some leader without question or taking a passive role in one's work setting, one's community, or one's professional organization will do little to advance the profession, promote individual growth, and achieve quality patient care. Instead, nursing needs followers who have characteristics that are similar to those of leaders: a willingness to serve, assertiveness, determination, a willingness to challenge ideas, courage, an ability to act as a change agent, and an openness to new ideas and perspectives. Indeed, followers and leaders must complement each other (Corona, 1986), as noted in Table 3–1.

Table 3–1	*Traits of Leaders and Followers*

Leaders	**Followers**
Study and create new ideas.	Test new ideas.
Make decisions.	Challenge decisions as needed.
Assign appropriate responsibilities.	Know when to accept responsibility and do so.
Create environments of trust, resulting in freedom.	Use freedom responsibly.
Take risks.	Risk following.
Are reliable.	Are trustworthy and respectful.
Are loyal to the followers.	Are loyal to the leader.
Are self-confident.	Know themselves.
Assume the leadership position.	Follow when appropriate.

Characteristics of Effective or Exemplary Followers

Although the term "follower" "conjures up images of docility, conformity, weakness, and failure to excel" (Chaleff, 1995, p. 3), effective or exemplary followers possess many of the same characteristics as those individuals who exercise leadership. Each of us may do well to reflect on the extent to which we are characterized by the following:

- Strength and independence
- Critical thinking
- An ability and willingness to think for ourselves
- An ability to give honest feedback and constructive criticism, particularly in a timely fashion
- A willingness to be our own person
- Innovativeness and creativity
- Active engagement in all we do

- Cooperativeness and collaborativeness
- A tendency to be a self-starter
- A tendency to "go above and beyond the call of duty"—to go beyond our job assignments
- A willingness to assume ownership
- A tendency to take initiative
- A positive sense of self-worth
- A "can do" aura (Kelley, 1992, p. 143)
- An attentiveness to what is happening around us
- A tendency to "hold up our end of the bargain"
- A sense of being energized by our work and the organization(s) in which we work

Through his work with workshop participants, Berg (1998) identified additional characteristics of exemplary followers. He described these individuals as "interesting characters" (p. 40) who were bold and colorful—not passive or bland—loyal, and supportive; they possessed their own distinctive voices that leaders typically heeded well. Exemplary followers openly expressed their own ideas, concerns, perspectives, and even conflicting views, and effective leaders paid attention to these voices. A nurse who proposes to the nurse manager and colleagues how family members can be more involved in planning and, indeed, coordinating or directing the care of patients with serious illnesses—when that is not the norm on the unit—is being bold, not passive, and expressing conflicting views. The colleagues who take this suggestion seriously and consider changing the practice standards on the unit are enriched by this nurse's proposal, and the ultimate goal toward which they are all working—quality patient and family care—is more likely to be realized.

Berg (1998) also found that an emotional connection exists between leaders and exemplary followers, a relation he suggested may be needed so that each can reassure the other "during those times when each must show his or her limits and weaknesses to the other" (p. 41). For example, the nurse manager who has been unsuccessful in securing additional staff positions so that nurses can attend valuable inservice programs and participate in grand rounds needs to be able to express that frustration. Likewise, staff need to be able to acknowledge when they do not have the knowledge or skill to care for a particular patient. Showing one's limitations and weaknesses requires a mutual trust, a bond, and an emotional connection between the leader and the followers.

> *"The secret of leadership is ... inviting cooperation from others, rather than demanding their obedience."*
>
> —J. Donald Walters

Effective followers, then, are far from invisible, and they are far from being clones of leaders. Instead, they actually stimulate and inspire leaders, challenge their creativity, collaborate with them, complement them, give them feedback, and support them. Leaders may inspire vision, but it is the followers who supply much of the energy to achieve that vision. Indeed, followership is "the important phenomenon to study if we are to understand why organizations succeed or fail" (Kelley, 1992, p. 5).

Followers assume such an active role, however, only when they get what they expect from leaders, and what they expect is credibility (Kouzes & Posner, 1993). Followers want leaders who are *honest*—individuals who are consistent, ethical, and principled. They want leaders who are *competent*—who know their field of endeavor and know the work that needs to be done. They want leaders who are *inspiring*—individuals who are enthusiastic, contagious, visionary, and effective in communicating a dream. And they want leaders who are *forward looking*—who are oriented toward the "big picture" and able to help followers see their important place in that picture. We might think of these factors in terms of a formula for successful leadership and for effective leader-follower relations:

Honesty + Competence + Inspiration + Vision = Credibility

Leaders and followers are therefore interdependent. Theirs is a reciprocal relationship, and they reinforce each other. Indeed, the qualities of leaders and followers are so closely aligned that one could assume that the same people who are seen by their peers as desirable leaders also would be seen as desirable followers. In addition, individuals often move back and forth between leader and follower roles, depending on the situation; they draw on the same skills to be effective in either role.

Although there are many opportunities for each of us to assume the role of leader, each of us also will have countless opportunities to function as a follower (Fig. 3–5). Therefore we consciously need to develop the skills of followership and cultivate and appreciate that role so that we can draw on those skills to assume the mantle of leadership when that becomes necessary.

Strategies to Develop Effective Followership Skills

In a commentary on heroes and brave men, Barbara Barnum (1987) noted that "sometimes a field, any field, needs a hero or a bunch of heroes, an elite to set its course, to chart new lands, to

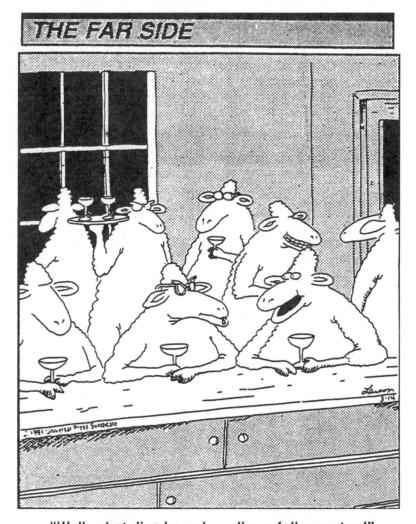

"Well, what d'ya know! . . . *I'm* a follower, too!"

Fig. 3–5 *The follower role is quite common.* (THE FAR SIDE © 1991 FARWORKS, INC.

brave new waters" (p. 5); the hero clears the way and "blazes the trail." Yet the only trails today's leaders can suggest, according to Barnum, "are slippery, fraught with rock slides, and inevitably lead up steep mountain sides" (p. 5), making it difficult for even the best of followers. Despite this challenge, however, in the contemporary world—and even more so in the future—the heroes may have the easier job and the followers the more difficult one.

Barnum asserted that "never before has the action of the masses had such potential to influence the direction of our profession" (1987, p. 5). It is the nurses who practice at the bedside who demonstrate what quality patient care is, not the administrator who writes standards of care. It is the nurse working in the community who can influence local legislators with personalized human stories about the pain and suffering associated with polluted environments, lack of food and adequate shelter, and poor prenatal care, not the statisticians who merely cite numbers and trends without providing a human dimension. In other words, it is the followers who have the most significant impact on the future of our profession and the world, an idea supported by Vaclav Havel, the dissident who advocated solidarity in Communist Czechoslovakia and who asserted and demonstrated that "followers hold significant power, even in totalitarian states, . . . if they act on it" (Kelley, 1992, p. 235).

If it is true that the future of our profession and, indeed, the world will be most significantly affected by the actions of followers, then each of us needs to develop effective skills of followership, a notion expressed by many (Chaleff, 1995, 1998; DiRienzo, 1994; Guidera & Gilmore, 1988; Kelley, 1992, 1998; Litzinger & Schaefer, 1984; Lundy, 1993; Pittman, Rosenbach, & Potter, 1998). But how can we develop such skills? According to Chaleff (1998, p. 89), "follower skills are learned informally, like street fighting," but they are, nevertheless, learned.

In a recent book on "paths to leadership," Andersen (1999) does not talk about followers or followership, per se. However, she and the various contributing authors do talk about how students can chart a course toward assuming leadership positions in nursing. Inherent in those discussions is an implication that one develops as a leader by being an effective follower, a strategy Kelley (1992) refers to as "apprenticeship." Indeed, Aristotle, Plato, Homer, Hegel, and the military academy at West Point, among others, insist that mastering followership is a necessary part of becoming an effective leader (Kelley, 1992; Rosenbach & Taylor, 1998).

Thus, one of the strategies suggested for nurses who aspire to effective followership and leadership is to apprentice yourself as a follower by assuming that role, thinking about what it means, reflecting on how you are contributing to your organization and the nursing profession by fulfilling that role, and *being the best you can be.* In addition, you would do well to study and implement many of the strategies that are suggested (later in this text and elsewhere) for developing leaders because those roles are so complementary. Among the strategies that may be used to help you be a more effective or exemplary follower are the following:

- Continue your education, both formal and informal. Knowledge is power and will serve you well as a follower.
- Be involved in your practice setting. Have a sense of ownership and stewardship; do not be merely a spectator.
- Take initiative. Take action without being told to do so.
- Be committed to something other than your own career development. Find your passion in life, and be passionate about what you do.
- Know your organization.
- Know your own values and hold on to them.
- Set a standard that demonstrates high values. Others will model that.
- When they impede progress, be willing to "bend, circumvent, or break the rules to get things done" (Chaleff, 1995, p. 47).
- Be involved in professional organizations.
- Seek mentors or accept an offer of mentoring if it is made.
- Develop your professional networks—within and outside your organization —and use them.
- Accept a place at the table where decisions are made, or if such a place is not offered, create such a place for yourself. For example, agree to serve on a committee when invited to do so or volunteer to revise the admission data form if the one currently being used focuses too much on patient weaknesses and limitations and does not adequately address patient strengths and abilities.
- Feel free to criticize, but do not just complain and walk away.
- Be proactive. Advocate and be a catalyst for change.
- Remain fully accountable for your actions.
- Share information rather than hoard it.
- Help colleagues grow and do their job well. Help them develop the skills of giving needed feedback.
- Be reflective.
- Have a sense of humor and laugh at your own mistakes.
- Develop positive relationships with colleagues, rely on each other, and be responsible to each other. Be a good team player.
- Continue to develop a wide array of skills, including communication skills, assertiveness skills, clinical practice skills, decision-making skills, and writing skills.
- Analyze your own performance by asking others for feedback and being honest in your own self-appraisal. Do you engage in gossip? Do you use language that suggests you are not as important as other people or your ideas and suggestions are not as valuable as theirs? Do you allow yourself

to be subservient? Are you cynical? Do you allow the leader or others to show disrespect for your coworkers' ideas or views? Are you willing to take risks? Are you destructive when you offer criticism?

- Contribute as an equal partner.
- Independently think up and champion new ideas.
- Try to solve difficult problems rather than expecting the leader to do it all.
- Figure out the steps that are needed for the group to achieve its goals, then be sure to be an integral part of those steps rather than on the periphery of "the action."
- Be cooperative with, rather than adversarial to, the leader.
- Appreciate the needs, goals, and constraints placed on the leader.
- Play devil's advocate.
- Give credit where it is due.
- Follow through on your commitments. Be credible.
- Know your job and do it well. Be competent, demonstrate your value to the group, and make a difference to the organization.
- Exercise a "courageous conscience . . . the ability to judge right from wrong and the fortitude to take affirmative steps toward what [you] believe is right" (Kelley, 1992, p. 168).
- Be enthusiastic and spread that enthusiasm to others.
- Know yourself and be honest with yourself.
- Be comfortable with uncertainty and ambiguity. Resist the understandable fear of the unknown.
- Seek wise counsel.
- Speak up so others can benefit from your views. Speak the truth and be willing to "stand up, to stand out, to risk rejection, to initiate conflict" (Chaleff, 1995, p. 7).
- Present your position in a forthright manner. Develop excellence in communication by using a variety of channels.
- Develop self confidence. Believe in and have faith in yourself.
- Remain calm. Do not be hostile.
- "Discover or create opportunities to fulfill [your] potential and maximize [your] value to the organization" (Chaleff, 1995, p. 6).
- Provide opportunities for the leader to talk about his or her vulnerabilities and concerns, as well as his or her strengths and vision.
- Help sacred cows be "gently led to pasture" (Chaleff, 1995, p. 89) so that all subjects are open to discussion and all options are possible. Do not discard what may seem like wild ideas before considering them carefully.
- Develop a record of successes.

- Do deep breathing or other relaxation exercises before having a conversation with an authority figure.
- Do not give in to peer pressure.
- Ask for feedback.
- Set personal goals and take responsibility to meet them.
- Stand up for and support your leader when he or she needs to make difficult decisions.
- Ask a great deal of the leader, but do not expect perfection from him or her.
- Express skepticism about ideas, proposals, and "pronouncements," but do so in a respectful way.
- "Learn the ropes," "pay your dues," and prove yourself in the follower role.
- Be dependable and reliable.
- Be creative.
- "Refuse to be used and abused" (Barron, 1998, p. 2).

It is obvious that there are many ways in which you can be an effective or exemplary follower. It also is obvious that it is only with concerted personal effort that you will develop the skills of effective followership. These "keys to effective followership" may be summarized in many ways, but the listing offered by Barron (1998, p. 2) seems to "say it all:"

- Be a critical thinker, not a "yes" person.
- Be consistent and dependable.
- Be humble and patient.
- Be able to receive and offer constructive criticism.
- Be a tireless worker.
- Be a disciplined student of study and work (theory and practice).
- Be persistent and consistent at developing leadership (and followership) skills.
- Be a thinker!
- Be a thinker!!
- Be a thinker!!!

CONCLUSION

Leadership and followership have an equal influence on each other. They exist side by side, and one is not more important than the other. Indeed, the "connections between what were previously thought to be separate entities" (Wheatley, 1992, p. 10)—leadership and followership—are significant.

Followers have more power than they may realize. They confer the leadership role, and "the responsibility for making the leader-follower relationship work remains with the 'follower'" (Berg, 1998, p. 33). Indeed, followers can create a "conspiracy" (Bennis, 1989) that, although largely unconscious, can prevent leaders from leading, keeping them from "taking charge and making changes" (p. xii). "We are a nation of followers" (Kelley, 1992, p. 24), where "the spirit of American democracy elevates and celebrates the role of the follower" (p. 24). In such a society, the masses actually create history, and because "healthy followership is a conscious act of free will" (Chaleff, 1995, p.151), the masses allow certain individuals to exert leadership. Leaders, then, are accountable to followers, and followers play a significant role.

All of us are both leaders and followers, and most of us are followers more than we are leaders. That, however, is not anything for which we should apologize or anything about which we should feel badly. "Leaders cannot function without the eyes and ears and minds and hearts of followers" (DePree, 1992, p. 200), and they "only really accomplish something by permission of the followers" (p. 201). "The mark of a great leader is the development and growth of followers. The mark of a great follower is the growth of leaders" (Chaleff, 1995, p. 27). Therefore, instead of feeling insignificant in the role of follower, we should rejoice!

Critical Thinking 3-1

Critical Thinking Exercises

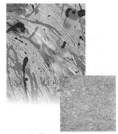

What is appealing about being in the follower role?
What is unattractive about being in that role?

_____

_____

_____

Review the characteristics of effective followers. How would you describe yourself in the follower role? How effective have you been in that role?

_____

_____

Talk to your nursing colleagues about followership. What are their views on the concept? Was the concept ever addressed in their educational programs? Do they rate themselves as effective followers? How did they develop the abilities to be effective in that role? Whom do they identify as the most effective followers among their work group? What is the basis for that rating? Are these the same individuals they identify as leaders (or potential leaders) among the group?

_____

_____

How do your colleagues' opinions on followership and its development compare with your own views? How are nurses' views similar to or different from those outside healthcare or those outside a predominantly female field?

_____

_____

Should we perhaps focus more on developing enlightened followers in nursing than on developing leaders all around us?

Read Chaleff's (1995, pp. 177–178) "Meditation on Followership." Are these principles by which you could live and that could guide your practice as a follower? This meditation may be something to review regularly as you implement your role as a professional nurse.

"*Meditation on Followership*"

by Chaleff

I am a steward of this group and share responsibility for its success.
I am responsible for adhering to the highest values I can envision.
I am responsible for my successes and failures and for continuing to learn from them.
I am responsible for the attractive and unattractive parts of who I am.
I can empathize with others who are also imperfect.
As an adult, I can relate on a peer basis to other adults who are the group's formal leaders.
I can support leaders and counsel them, and receive support and counsel from them.
Our common purpose is our best guide.
I have the power to help leaders use their power wisely and effectively.
If leaders abuse power, I can help them change their behavior.
If I abuse power, I can learn from others and change my behavior.
If abusive leaders do not change their behavior, I can and will withdraw my support.
By staying true to my values, I can serve others well and fulfill my potential.
Thousands of courageous acts by followers can, one by one, improve the world.
Courage always exists in the present. What can I do today?

Complete the following "Followership Style Test." What did you learn about yourself by taking this test? What did you learn about followership and the relationship between followers and leaders?

Followership Style Test

This questionnaire includes statements about the type of boss you prefer. Imagine yourself to be in a subordinate position of some kind and use your responses to indicate your preference for the way in which a leader might relate with you.

The format includes a five-point scale rating from "Strongly Agree" to "Strongly Disagree" for each statement. Select one point on each scale and mark it as you read the 16 statements relating to followership.

	SA	A	MF	D	SD
1. I expect my job to be very explicitly outlined for me.	1	2	3	4	5
2. When the boss says to do something, I do it. After all, he or she is the boss.	1	2	3	4	5
3. Rigid rules and regulations usually cause me to become frustrated and inefficient.	5	4	3	2	1
4. I am ultimately responsible for and capable of self-discipline based on my contacts with the people around me.	5	4	3	2	1
5. My jobs should be made as short in duration as possible so that I can achieve efficiency through repetition.	1	2	3	4	5
6. Within reasonable limits I will try to accommodate requests from persons who are not my boss because these requests are typically in the best interests of the company anyway.	5	4	3	2	1
7. When the boss tells me to do something that is the wrong thing to do, it is his or her fault, not mine, when I do it.	1	2	3	4	5
8. It is up to my leader to provide a set of rules by which I can measure my performance.	1	2	3	4	5
9. The boss is the boss. And the fact of the promotion suggests that he or she has something on the ball.	1	2	3	4	5
10. I accept orders only from my boss.	1	2	3	4	5
11. I would prefer for my boss to give me general objectives and guidelines and then allow me to do the job my way.	5	4	3	2	1
12. If I do something that is not right, it is my own fault, even if my supervisor told me to do it.	5	4	3	2	1
13. I prefer jobs that are not repetitive, the kind of task that is new and different each time.	5	4	3	2	1

SA = Strongly agree; A = agree; MF = mixed feelings; D = disagree; SD = strongly disagree.

	SA	A	MF	D	SD
14. My supervisor is in no way superior to me by virtue of positions. He or she does a different kind of job, one that includes a lot of managing and coordinating.	5	4	3	2	1
15. I expect my leader to give me disciplinary guidelines.	1	2	3	4	5
16. I prefer to tell my supervisor what I will or at least should be doing. I am ultimately responsible for my own work.	5	4	3	2	1

SA = Strongly agree; A = agree; MF = mixed feelings; D = disagree; SD = strongly disagree.

Scoring

Score your own followership style by simply averaging the numbers for your answers to the individual items. For example, if you scored item number one "Strongly Agree," you will find the point value of "1" for that answer. To obtain your overall followership style, add all the numerical values that are associated with the 16 followership items and divide by 16. The resulting average is your followership style.

Score	Description	Followership Style
≤1.9	Very autocratic	Cannot function well without programs and procedures; needs feedback
2.0–2.4	Moderately autocratic	Needs solid structure and feedback but can also carry on independently
2.5–3.4	Mixed	Mixture of above and below
3.5–4.0	Moderately participative	Independent worker, does not need close supervision, just a bit of feedback
≥4.1	Very democratic	Self-starter, likes to challenge new things by himself or herself

Source: *Adapted from* Douglas, L.M. (1992). *The effective nurse leader and manager* (4th ed.) (pp. 25–28). St. Louis: Mosby.

References

Anderson, C.A. (1999). *Nursing student to nursing leader: The critical path to leadership development.* Albany, NY: Delmar.

Barnum, B. (1987). The need for heros [sic] and the need for brave men. *Courier (Newsletter of the Teachers College, Columbia University Nursing Education Alumni Association) 54,* 5.

Barron, C. (1998). *Dare to lead.* www.dynamicleadership.com/leader.html (January 26, 1998).

Bennis, W. (1989). *Why leaders can't lead. The unconscious conspiracy continues.* San Francisco: Jossey-Bass.

Berg, D.N. (1998). Resurrecting the muse. Followership in organizations. In E.B. Klein, F. Gabelnick, & P. Herr (Eds.), *The psychodynamics of leadership* (pp. 27–52). Madison, CT: Psychosocial Press.

Brown, B. (1980). Follow the leader. *Nursing Outlook 28*(6), 357–359.

Chaleff, I. (1998). Learn the art of followership. In W.E. Rosenbach & R.L. Taylor (Eds.), *Contemporary issues in leadership* (4th ed.) (pp. 89–91). Boulder, CO: Westview Press.

Chaleff, I. (1995). *The courageous follower. Standing up to and for our leaders.* San Francisco: Berrett-Koehler.

Corona, D. (1986). Followership: The indispensable corollary to leadership. In E.C. Hein & M.J. Nicholson (Eds.), *Contemporary leadership behavior: Selected readings* (2nd ed.) (pp. 87–91). Boston: Little, Brown.

DePree, M. (1992). *Leadership jazz.* New York: Doubleday Currency.

DiRienzo, S.M. (1994). A challenge to nursing: Promoting followers as well as leaders. *Holistic Nursing Practice 9*(1), 26–30.

Dreher, D. (1996). *The Tao of personal leadership.* New York: HarperBusiness.

Guidera, M.K., & Gilmore, C. (1988). In defense of followership. *American Journal of Nursing 88*(7), 1017.

Joel, L.A. (1999). Life review of an ANA President: The path of leadership. In C.A. Andersen (Ed.), *Nursing student to nursing leader: The critical path to leadership development* (pp. 17–32). Albany, NY: Delmar.

Kelley, R. (1992). *The power of followership: How to create leaders people want to follow and followers who lead themselves.* New York: Doubleday Currency.

Kelley, R.E. (1998). In praise of followers. In W.E. Rosenbach & R.L. Taylor (Eds.), *Contemporary issues in leadership* (4th ed.) (pp. 96–106). Boulder, CO: Westview Press.

Kouzes, J.M., & Posner, B.Z. (1993). *Credibility: How leaders gain and lose it. Why people demand it.* San Francisco: Jossey-Bass.

Litzinger, W., & Schaefer, T. (1984). Leadership through followership. In W.E. Rosenbach & R.L. Taylor (Eds.), *Contemporary issues in leadership* (pp. 138–143). Boulder, CO: Westview Press.

Lundy, J.L. (1993). *Lead, follow, or get out of the way. Invaluable insights into leadership styles.* San Diego: Pfeiffer & Co.

O'Neil, E., & Coffman, J. (Eds.). (1998). *Strategies for the future of nursing: Changing roles, responsibilities, and employment patterns of registered nurses.* San Francisco: Jossey-Bass.

Pittman, T.S., Rosenbach, W.E., & Potter, E.H., III. (1998). Followers as partners: Taking the initiative for action. In W.E. Rosenbach & R.L. Taylor (Eds.), *Contemporary issues in leadership* (4th ed.) (pp. 107–120). Boulder, CO: Westview Press.

Porter-O'Grady, T. (1993). Of mythspinners and mapmakers: 21st century managers. *Nursing Management 24*(4), 52–55.

Rocchiccioli, J.T., & Tilbury, M.S. (1998). *Clinical leadership in nursing.* Philadelphia: Saunders.

Rosenbach, W.E., & Taylor, R.L. (1998). Followership: The underappreciated dimension. In W.E. Rosenbach & R.L. Taylor (Eds.), *Contemporary issues in leadership* (4th ed.) (pp. 85–88). Boulder, CO: Westview Press.

Staub, R.E., II. (1996). *The heart of leadership: 12 practices of courageous leaders.* Provo, UT: Executive Excellence Publishing.

Sullivan, T.J. (1998). *Collaboration: A health care imperative.* New York: McGraw-Hill.

Swansburg, R.C., & Swansburg, R.J. (1999). *Introductory management and leadership for nurses* (2nd ed.). Sudbury, MA: Jones & Bartlett.

Wheatley, M.J. (1992). *Leadership and the new science. Learning about organization from an orderly universe.* San Francisco: Berrett-Koehler.

Yoder-Wise, P.S. (1999). *Leading and managing in nursing* (2nd ed.). St. Louis: Mosby.

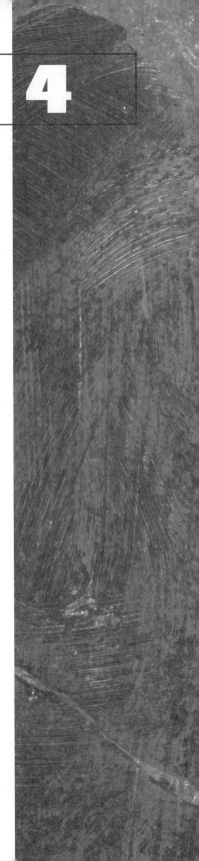

CHAPTER 4

Leadership as an Integral Component of a Professional

Leadership as an Integral Component of a Professional

Learning Objectives

☐ Identify characteristics of transformational and transactional leaders.

☐ Compare and contrast the leader-follower relationship in a transformational environment and the leader-follower relationship in a transactional environment.

☐ Explain how transformational leadership generates growth in an individual, an organization, and a group.

☐ Describe how Maslow's hierarchy of needs relates to leadership development.

☐ Explain how leadership is an integral component of each professional nurse's role.

INTRODUCTION

Professional nurses can no longer think of themselves as "just nurses." Nurses are increasingly expected to provide leadership, whether they hold staff positions or are vice presidents, nurse practitioners, or nurse educators. Therefore it is important for all professional nurses to be self-confident, have a high degree of self-esteem, and be visionary. (See Chapter 5 for a discussion of vision.) Individuals with these strengths will be able to exert leadership in making decisions, facilitating partnerships with patients and other healthcare workers, accomplishing goals, and reaching stated visions.

When thinking about the leadership that is exercised in a nursing group or organization, it must be realized that every individual, not just the nurse manager or dean or committee chair, has the potential and the responsibility to assume the role of leader. The individual who happens to be in the appointed, authoritative role (e.g., the nurse manager) may or may not be the person who actually fulfills the role of the leader. As discussed earlier, effective followers have skills comparable to those of leaders, and the effectiveness of the leadership that any individual provides depends largely on the followers. Gardner (1990) said "leadership can be distributed among members and the leader must recognize the needs of the followers, help them see how these needs can be met, and give them confidence that they can accomplish the results through their own efforts" (p. 149). So leaders must be able to lead others as well as themselves. Then, and only if there is a determined and powerful followership, can leaders be successful. Hence, as strong followers, effective nurses actually are exerting leadership.

It is not uncommon, however, for nurses to fail to be effective followers or leaders. Consider the following situations: instead of acting as leaders or effective followers, nurses criticize their managers, the institutions, the director, the doctor, and other people occupying positions of leadership. Nurses "eat their young," blame other nurses, and fail to collaborate with each other. Nurses fail to challenge the "orders" of a physician, fail to capitalize on their extensive knowledge or experience, or claim to be "only a nurse" when talking to a physician or a patient. These examples point to a low self-esteem on the part of these nurses. If nurses are to increase their responsibility and if the profession is to survive and thrive, all nurses must exercise their leadership ability.

Leaders are not born leaders; rather, leaders emerge and continue to evolve as a result of experiences and interactions with a variety of people. All nurses need to practice their leadership and encourage others to get involved in leading either as a follower or as a leader. By creating a vision, strategizing how to accomplish the vision, seeking creative ways to implement change, and effectively leading or following in a collaborative manner, nurses can learn new leadership skills that will assist not only them but the entire healthcare team in accomplishing the goals.

Types of Leadership

Burns (1978) describes two types of leadership that leaders use to make change and create new futures: transactional leadership and transformational leadership.

TRANSACTIONAL LEADERSHIP

Transactional leadership involves an exchange in which both the leader and the followers "get something." The leader gets the job completed or the goal achieved, and the followers get promotions, money, or other benefits. The focus of this type of leadership system is the accomplishment of a task, a goal easily seen in many nursing situations. Some even argue that nurses focus too often on tasks. Transactional leaders focus on getting the job done and see task completion as the bottom line. Zaleznik (1989) characterized transactional leaders as manipulative, detached, and inscrutable. Although there may be some type of "connection" between these leaders and their followers, this connection often is something other than a common purpose or a shared vision. With such a relationship, both leaders and followers may perceive their work only as a job and not as a career.

TRANSFORMATIONAL LEADERSHIP

Transformational leadership is a process in which "leaders and followers raise one another to higher levels of motivation and morality" (Burns, 1978, p. 20). This motivation energizes people to perform beyond expectations by creating a sense of ownership in reaching the vision. Bass (1985, pp. 62, 67) compares transformational leadership with inspirational leadership that arouses motivation of followers. He cites examples of transformational leadership from a Reserve Officer Training Cadet (ROTC) study, including the following:

- Instilling pride in all
- Building morale through "pep talks"
- Acting as a positive role model
- Building the confidence of others through personal encouragement
- Complimenting individuals' performances and contributions as a way to instill pride in the group

Bass (1985) characterized transformational leaders as charismatic, able to instill motivation in others, and able to give individualized consideration; Burns (1978) described them as individuals who heighten followers' awareness of what must be done to accomplish the shared goal. Bennis and Nanus (1985, p. 3) defined transformational leaders as individuals who "commit people to action, who convert followers into leaders, and who convert leaders into agents of change."

> *"All great leaders have had one characteristic in common: it was the willingness to confront unequivocally the major anxiety of their people in their time."*
>
> —John Kenneth Gailbraith

Several strategies have been identified (Bennis & Nanus, 1985) to assist leaders to be more transformational: attention through vision, meaning through communication, trust through positioning, and deployment of self through positive self-regard and optimism about a desired outcome. In other words, nurses must pay more attention to emphasizing the importance of following a vision and assisting others to participate in making it a reality; nurses must communicate their values and beliefs to each other so that they can achieve a common meaning in their work and realize the vision toward which they are striving; nurses must trust others, be honest, and act responsibly; and finally, nurses must use their talents and expertise as a way to express their desire and commitment to a vision. If nurses are to be transformational leaders, they must follow their dreams, communicate in an articulate manner, be concerned with their own growth as well as the growth of their followers, establish trusting relationships, and identify their strengths and limitations. They also need to readily accept change and constantly seek new ways of doing things despite the risk (Bass, 1985, p. 105).

Bass (1985) and Burns (1978) believe that transformational leaders have strong personal value systems, and by sharing these values, they are able to affect and even change followers' beliefs. This occurs without needing to negotiate "what's in it for the follower." In essence, transformational leaders have a spirit that creates special leader-follower relationships and that promotes individual and group growth. In fact, this spirit, this feeling of mutual involvement, is of greater significance than any isolated task accomplishment.

Curtain (1997) described transformational leaders as exciting because they represent something worthwhile, and that "something worthwhile" attracts followers. These transformational leaders are also effective because they reinstill hope in a world (or healthcare system) that is uncertain, ambiguous, and constantly changing.

Transformational Leadership and Nursing Practice

Wolf, Boland, and Ankerman (1994) describe how a transformational model encompassing four different paradigm shifts assisted them to transform their "outdated organization" (pp. 51–52) at Shadyside Hospital in Pittsburgh, Pennsylvania, into a successful nurse-patient-physician driven model of practice. The four paradigms reflect what most nurses have been educated (formally or informally) to believe; however, the authors challenge each paradigm in light of today's reality:

- "Nursing practice must evolve from a needs-driven model of care to one that is sensitive to limited resources" (p. 51). Today it has become impossible to fulfill every patient's needs. Nurses must contract with patients and payers to develop the most realistic plan of care for providing healthcare to each individual.
- "Nurses believe that there is a direct correlation between manpower and quality" (p. 52). More is not necessarily better; rather, it is the quality of the staff (as evidenced by their clinical competence and their ability to critically think through a problem and generate a decision) that is significant to provide high-quality patient care.
- "Standardization and routines for patient care will be replaced by individualization and creativity" (p. 52). Every intervention must be outcome-related and research-based.
- "Accountability, responsibility, and authority for clinical decision making will evolve from the manager to the practitioner, in partnership with the patient" (p. 52). Essentially all care provided by physicians and nurses must be negotiated with the individual patient, and nurses and patients, as well as physicians, must be active participants in planning and evaluating care.

These concepts are the cornerstones of the transformational model developed in this institution that gives leaders and followers opportunities to practice transformational leadership. The administrators and staff of Shadyside Hospital, who developed the model, also wanted all staff to depict four additional concepts (numbers 1 through 4) and their organization to depict three additional concepts (numbers 5 through 7):

1. *Hardiness,* which characterizes committed individuals who have a strong work ethic
2. *Empowerment,* which indicates individuals' abilities to feel confident about their strengths and realize the significance of their contributions
3. *Vision,* which drives one to accomplish a dream
4. *Decentralization,* which allows the "grass roots" of an organization to make decisions and delegate work
5. *Participative management,* which expects employees to be part of the decision-making process
6. An *organizational culture* that encompasses the values and beliefs the organization wants to promote
7. An *operating system* or structure that allows organizational goals to be accomplished

It is important to understand that the first four concepts must be present for the transformational model to be successful. The management concepts (numbers 5 through 7) would need to be conducive to creating unity and collaboration between workers, a holistic care approach, and a measurable patient outcome focus to care. Of course, the successful system must also be cost-efficient, provide high-quality care, and provide access to primary through tertiary care for a large number of individuals.

Self-Esteem and Leadership Image

Barker (1990) believes the most significant tool for transformational leaders to be effective is oneself, particularly one's self-awareness and self-development (p. 159). She clarifies this as a positive self-regard, which is what Bennis and Nanus (1985) delineate as a transformational leader. Barker (1990) and Burns (1978) recommend Maslow's (1970) explanation of esteem needs to better understand the concept of positive self-regard. Self-esteem includes the need for achievement, mastery, competence, confidence, independence, and freedom to act. Satisfying one's self-esteem needs tends to result in "self-confidence, worth, strength, capability, adequacy, and being useful and necessary" (Barker, 1990, p. 159). These abilities all correspond to a transformational leader and follower. Maslow's framework of hierarchical needs can be used to understand how leaders and followers develop. Individuals who have high self-esteem are able to develop and grow; followers can become leaders. This process of fulfilling needs assists the individual in acquiring leadership ability.

One must be self-motivated to change or improve one's situation in all aspects of life—personal and professional. Individuals who are not motivated to change will most likely remain at status quo and be unable to lead or facilitate others' growth. However, one should not expect success simply because one feels that he or she has worked very hard. A good example of this entitlement issue is depicted in the story (see Box 4–1) of an aspiring pre-Olympian who is not a transformational leader because she is so self-oriented (Campbell, 1996, p. 9).

Many nurses have the attitude that they expect better because they have seniority or have "paid their dues," and they allow themselves to be victims of the system. Things do not change just because people think they deserve special (different from the system constraints) favors; this only propagates more unhappiness for the nurse. One cannot allow oneself to be victimized.

Kouzes and Posner (1995) note that the unprecedented instability in today's world calls for strong leadership. They recommend that leaders engage in practices that transform followers and help realize visions:

- Challenge the status quo.
- Inspire a shared vision.
- Enable others to act, rather than to react.
- Be role models.
- Encourage the heart.

The first four practices are self-explanatory. The last practice, "encouraging the heart," is meant to highlight the importance of leaders caring deeply about their vision and working to accomplish the vision. It also advocates that people who perform well will be self-satisfied. Kouzes and Posner recommend that "leaders celebrate accomplishments," which makes a person "feel like a hero" (1995, p. 318). Perhaps it is more crucial as we enter the twenty-first century to garner more initiative, self-esteem, and assertiveness because many nursing professionals need to gain a higher positive self-regard. Nurses have been "controlled by forces outside themselves that had greater prestige, power, and status" (Roberts, 1983, p. 21); we have, in essence, allowed ourselves to be exploited.

Would-Be Leaders Become Leaders

Bennis (1993) explained the process of reinventing himself "to avoid accepting roles [which he] was brought up to play" (p. xv). He further described the significance of being able to invent and reinvent himself so he would not to have to be "content with borrowed postures, secondhand ideas, [or] fitting in instead of

Box 4–1 *Expect Success through Self-Confidence, Not Entitlement*

"One young lady had listed everything she had done to get into the finals, all of her exercising, her nutritional plans, her workouts, all of the sweat and pain and exertion and self-denial that she had gone through, and then she had written, "DESERVE a place on the Olympic team!" I [as her coach] had to take her aside and give her a short lecture about that kind of thinking.

"Look, I said. You don't deserve squat. Every other person in these trials has done exactly what you have done—they have exercised, they have sweated, they have gone through pain, they have given up other pleasures, they are just as deserving as you are. Saying that you deserve something special puts you in the role of potential victim, so that you can later say, Poor me, life has failed me."

"I told her, you can say I EXPECT to earn a place on the Olympic team. That's okay, that's an expression of self-confidence, a stance from where you can perform better because you expect to be among the best, but let's not have any more of these victimizing statements."

Source: Campbell, D. (1996). Inklings. *Issues & Observations 16*(1), 9.

standing out" (p. xv). Bennis warns us not to accept the stereotypical perception of what many nurses and nonnurses have perceived nursing to be. By reinventing oneself he is saying, "Do not accept the roles we were brought up to play"(Bennis, 1993, p. 2). Perhaps nurses as a group need to reinvent themselves and focus on larger issues rather than merely the tasks of the day. Nurses with tunnel vision tend to act as "passive followers," not as leaders, and to remain in positions in the organization that are less powerful (Kirchbaum, 1997, p. 12).

It is difficult to change one's perceptions about a role or the meaning of a specific profession's goal when one is entrenched in the role of carrying out another profession's orders. However, it is imperative that nurses begin to visualize that nursing is separate from medicine and that nursing is necessary for the greater good of healthcare. Kirchbaum (1997) suggests that "nurse educators include in their nursing leadership and management course the idea of helping students realize their knowledge, that personal power, those abilities they possess which contribute to solving a problem or accomplishing their goals" (p.12) is significant to the provision of high-quality care. It is imperative for nursing educators to foster leadership as an integral component of each nurse's role. Leadership skills must be deemed to be as important as the acquisition of clinical skills.

Leadership as an Integral Component of Each Nurse's Role

As the twenty-first century begins, nurses will increasingly be expected to assume the roles of advocate, teacher, caregiver, generator, disseminator of knowledge, manager, contributor to public health policy development, and leader. Nurses also will be expected to be heavily involved in partnering with other nurses and with representatives from all healthcare disciplines (*Nursing Leadership in the 21st Century*, 1996). Nurses in the twenty-first century must play a major role in evoking change in healthcare and work to ensure a significant role in the restructured system of managed care.

Nurses must acquire principle-centered leadership to be leaders in the new healthcare system. Principle-centered leadership involves "keeping promises, developing virtues, changing bad habits, being faithful to vows, exercising courage, and being genuinely considerate of others" (Covey, 1991, p. 18). These principles are similar to compasses in that they always point the way and keep us from becoming lost amid conflicting ideas and values. Covey (1991) says principles constantly apply and they surface in the form of "ideas, norms, values, and teachings which uplift, fulfill, empower, and inspire people" (p. 19). Characteristics that exemplify principle-centered leaders include continually learning, service orientation, having positive energy, believing in others, leading a balanced life, viewing life as an adventure, being synergistic, and having the ability to self-renew (p. 33).

Leaders-to-be must develop communication skills because this is paramount to being an effective leader. It is necessary for nurses to be consistent, assertive, and knowledgeable speakers about their role, the state of current healthcare, and their patients' care. Likewise, it is mandatory for nurses to have sophisticated interpersonal relationship skills with patients and their families or significant others.

Credibility is another important characteristic that admired leaders possess. Kouzes and Posner (1993, p. 50) studied people's reasons for respecting, trusting, and being willing to be influenced by others and found the following commonly cited behaviors as indicative of credibility: supported me, had the courage to do the right thing, challenged me, developed and acted as a mentor to others, listened, celebrated good work, followed through on commitments, trusted me, empowered others, made time for people, shared the vision, opened doors, overcame personal hardships, admitted mistakes, advised others, solved problems creatively, and taught well. These behaviors reflect the characteristics of a transformational leader. The four components that correlated highest with being credible included honesty, competency, inspiration, and being forward-looking (Kouzes & Posner, 1993).

> *"To achieve all that is possible, we must attempt the impossible ... to be as much as we can be, we must dream of being more."*
> —Gale Baker Stanton

Leaders must also engage in self-renewal or reinvention of self. The ability to evaluate where one is in one's life and plan how to get to the place where one wants to be takes leadership. Of course, it would be far easier to accept the status quo and just "float" personally and professionally through one's life. It would be far more productive and self-actualizing to develop a clear idea of one's vision and work toward accomplishing it.

Taking a risk to try something new, taking time to dream and imagine how one could make a difference, joining a professional organization and getting actively involved on a committee, and taking a noncredit course, such as public speaking, or credit-bearing courses toward the completion of a degree or a certificate all are activities that people should consider. By self-evaluating or using peer evaluation consistently, one can identify strengths and weaknesses. Hence people can nurture their strengths and either work on their limitations or work around them. Nurses can also gather their strengths and "learn to learn while doing" (Margerison & Kakabadse, 1984, p. 24). So many of us believe we have to be competent in anything we undertake and therefore generally do not take a promotion or transfer to another nursing unit because we feel it is safer to maintain what we already do "best."

As leaders in the healthcare arena today, nurses must embody all of the aforementioned for nursing services to be accessible to patients, for nurses to be involved in multidisciplinary collaboration, and for nursing care to be identified as the reason for positive and cost-effective patient outcomes. Nurses must spearhead new health promotion strategies that provide measurable and successful patient outcomes.

In his book *Seven Habits of Highly Effective People: Conveying a Leadership Image,* Covey (1989) summarized how would-be leaders can become more effective leaders by using his seven habits. Those habits are as follows: be proactive, begin with the end (goal) in mind, put first things first, think win/win, seek first to understand—then to be understood, synergize, and sharpen the saw (be proactive about the future).

As leaders, we are incredibly visible, and the image we convey can have a significant impact on the way we are perceived by others, the way in which others respond to us, and our ultimate effectiveness. What we say, how we say it, how we look, and what and how we write all are means by which an image is conveyed. No matter how competent we are, if we do not convey a leadership image, it is unlikely we will be successful leaders.

Davis (1991) says that 55 percent of what people believe is obtained visually. Trust in a leader will be built by positive verbal and visual imaging, as well as how a leader relates to followers. It is therefore imperative for nurses to attend to all aspects of their "general presence" because this will either impress their colleagues or fail to leave a lasting impression. It is important for nurses to project themselves as knowledgeable in all types of forums, most especially multidisciplinary collaboration.

CONCLUSION

One does not have to be in nursing management to be a "true" nursing leader. This has overwhelming implications for nurses. It is time for nurses to realize their potential and reinvent themselves. As Bennis (1993, p. 1) recommended, "people who cannot reinvent themselves must be content with borrowed postures, secondhand ideas, and fitting in instead of standing out." Nurses are increasingly "standing out" as they begin new roles in promoting health in inner-city homeless centers and school-based health clinics or taking healthcare vans to the most needy of people. Nurses are starting satellite outpatient dialysis and chemotherapy centers, cardiac rehabilitation centers, and preoperative learning clinics to assist people in restoring their health. Nurses in acute-care areas are developing new nurse-driven protocols, collaborating with other healthcare disciplines in creating critical pathways that focus patient care on meeting outcomes, and participating in teaching smoking cessation, cholesterol lowering, and alternative nonpharmacological programs. Many transformational nursing leaders are making a difference in patient outcomes, as well as using their leadership potential to meet their own expectations of self. Nursing educators must revise curricula to provide students opportunities to practice as much leadership as clinical skills. Nurses also must learn how to mentor each other to facilitate a stronger front, much like flocks of birds who fly in a V formation to strengthen their flying range (see Box 4–2).

Box 4–2 *Learning Lessons from Geese*

Although we may know that geese fly in a V formation, what we may not know is that as each bird flaps its wings, it creates an uplift for the bird following. By flying in formation, the whole flock adds 71 percent more to the flying range than if each bird flew alone.

A second fact about geese is that when the lead goose gets tired, it moves back into the formation and another goose flies the point position.

Third, if a goose falls out of the formation, it feels the drag and resistance of trying to fly alone and quickly gets back into formation to take advantage of the power of the bird it follows.

What are the lessons here for leadership? First, leadership must be shared; we all must take our turn doing the work that will help our profession evolve, our organizations grow, and ourselves continue to develop. Second, every member of the group has the potential to "fly the point position" and serve as the leader; we should not limit our expectations of the potential within each of us. Finally, the work we do can stimulate and excite others in our group to also perform better and achieve a level of excellence perhaps unexpected previously. Indeed, there is much we can learn about leaders and leadership from geese. We need only to pay attention and be open to new ideas, perspectives, and possibilities.

Critical Thinking 4–1

Critical Thinking Exercises

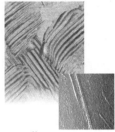

Describe how you could reinvent yourself, personally and professionally, so as not to merely "live the status quo." _____

_____

_____

Reflect on Covey's seven habits of highly effective people and brainstorm on how you could incorporate them into your nursing practice.

_____

_____

How would you describe the image of individuals you think of as leaders? individuals you do not consider to be leaders? What are some of the differences between those two groups of individuals in terms of a "leadership image"?

_____

_____

How would you describe the image you convey? Look at the way you dress, things you have written, presentations you have made, your participation on committees or in class, and so on. Is this the kind of image you want to convey? If not, what aspects are unsatisfactory to you, and how could you change them?

_____

_____

Compare the "leadership image" of nurses in various roles: staff nurse, advanced practice nurse, nurse educator, nursing service administrator, and so on. How are they alike? How are they different? What kinds of things can a nurse do to convey a strong image?

_____

_____

What can aspiring nurse leaders do to overcome negative stereotypes of nurses and nursing, create a genuinely positive leadership image, and convey that image to achieve desired goals?

_____

_____

References

Barker, A. (1990). *Transformational nursing leadership: A vision for the future.* Baltimore: Williams & Wilkins.

Bass, B. (1985). *Leadership and performance beyond expectations.* New York: Macmillan.

Bennis, W. (1993). *An invented life: Reflections on leadership and change.* Reading, MA: Addison-Wesley.

Bennis, W., & Nanus, B. (1985). *Leadership: The strategies for taking charge.* New York: Harper & Row.

Burns, J. (1978). *Leadership.* New York: Harper & Row.

Campbell, D. (1996). Inklings. *Issues & Observations 16*(1), 9.

Covey, S. (1991). *Principle-centered leadership.* New York: Summit Books.

Covey, S. (1989). *Seven habits of highly effective people.* New York: Fireside.

Curtain, L. (1997). How and how not to be a transformational leader. *Nursing Management 28*(2), 7–8.

Davis, C. (1991). Dress for success. *Nursing Spectrum*, March 25, 1991.

Gardner, J. (1990). *On leadership.* New York: Free Press.

Kirchbaum, K. (1997). Preparing students for leadership in practice. *Creative Nursing 3*(2), 12–14.

Kouzes, J., & Posner, B. (1995). *The leadership challenge: How to keep getting extraordinary things done in organizations* (2nd ed.). San Francisco: Jossey-Bass.

Kouzes, J., & Posner, B. (1993). *Credibility: How leaders gain and lose it, why people demand it.* San Francisco: Jossey-Bass.

Margerison, C., & Kakabadse, A. (1984). *How American chief executives succeed.* New York: American Management Association.

Maslow, A. (1970). *Motivation and personality* (2nd ed.). New York: Harper & Row.

Nursing leadership in the 21st century (ARISTA II Conference Proceedings). (1996). Indianapolis: Sigma Theta Tau International.

Roberts, S. (1983). Oppressed group behavior: Implications for nursing. *Advances in Nursing Science 5*(4), 21–30.

Wolf, G., Boland, S., & Ankerman, M. (1994). A transformational model for the practice of professional nursing. Part 1. *Journal of Nursing Administration 24*(4), 51–57.

Zaleznik, A. (1989). *The managerial mystique: Restoring leadership in business.* New York: Harper & Row.

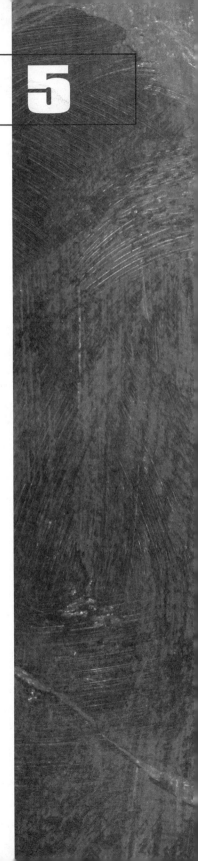

CHAPTER **5**

Vision and Creativity

Vision and Creativity

Learning Objectives

- ☐ Define the concept of vision as it relates to leadership.
- ☐ Describe how a nurse leader or follower can facilitate the identification, articulation, and communication of a personal vision.
- ☐ Identify strategies that would be effective in making one's personal vision become a reality.
- ☐ Formulate a personal vision for the profession or one's particular area of practice.
- ☐ Identify characteristics of nursing and nonnursing leaders who are viewed as visionary.
- ☐ Describe characteristics of a creative person, process, and environment.
- ☐ Project potential outcomes of using creativity as a nurse leader or follower.
- ☐ Identify how the new science of leadership fosters an individual's creativity in order to improve leadership and followership.
- ☐ Examine how the incorporation of vision and creativity into one's profession can help vitalize and energize a nurse.

INTRODUCTION

One of the most significant characteristics of a leader is to have a vision of a "better world." The 1990s have brought an abundance of words such as "vision," "impact," "empowerment," and "facilitation" to everyday conversation. As we move into the new century, however, the time has come to stop talking about the words and begin to take action.

Having and conveying a vision, as well as being able to energize followers to join in the effort of making that vision a reality, involves credibility, communication skills, an ability to maintain momentum, and creativity. Although nurses typically are skilled in communication, have high energy levels, and are seen as credible, they often do not think of themselves as creative and often have difficulty sustaining the momentum of a group. The mere idea of being creative may seem foreign to many nurses who are accustomed to following fairly strict protocols for delivering patient care. In addition, the expectation that nurses have and can articulate a vision also may seem unusual if one has been socialized to expect that only the chief executive officer (CEO) or vice president has the right or responsibility to advance a vision. Being able to incorporate the new philosophy of what leadership is into one's professional role, accepting responsibility for articulating a vision, and allowing oneself to be creative are essential for the nurse who will be practicing in the twenty-first century.

Leaders do many extraordinary things, but one of the greatest contributions they make is having a focus or a purpose that emerges from their knowledge and experience and that reflects their idea of what would better the group in question. As Bennis (1989, p. 30) says, "The first basic ingredient of leadership is a guiding vision." Indeed, "a leader without some vision of where he wants to take his organization is not a leader" (Bennis, 1989, p. 30). There are three major aspects of visionary leadership: the construction of the vision to encompass the image of an organization or group, the development of a set of strategies that make the vision a driving force for the organization or group, and the leader's ability to communicate the vision and engage every member of the organization or group in making it become a reality (Sashkin, 1989).

> *"Not much happens without a dream. Behind every great achievement is a dreamer of great dreams. Much more than a dream is required to bring it to reality; but the dream must be there first."*
>
> —Robert Greenleaf

The Concept of Vision

WHAT IS A VISION?

Visions are dreams or ideas that are "specific enough to provide guidance to people yet vague enough to encourage initiative and to remain relevant under a variety of conditions"
(Kotter, 1990, p. 36). A vision is also an image of where the organization or group wants to be in the future (Conger, 1989). A
vision is different from a goal because it is broad and it does
not focus on a "greater return of assets or increased market
share or introduction of a new product" (Conger, 1989, p. 38).
Kouzes and Posner (1993) studied 90 leaders in large organizations and found vision to be identified as a key strategy for
their success. Some of the participants described a vision as "a
purpose, mission, legacy, dream, goal, calling, and a personal
agenda" (p. 94). Conger (1989) believes that most visions can
be categorized into one of four types (Fig. 5–1): those with an
external orientation (e.g., a marketing innovation), those with
an internal orientation (e.g., a transformation of the organization's mission), those that are narrow in focus, and those that
are more broadly focused.

Obviously, a vision overlaps a variety of ideas and values in
an organization or group. It may begin with an internal orientation and a narrow perspective, and then grow into a more external direction with a broader perspective. In nursing, critical
pathways may be a step in realizing the vision to "refocus care

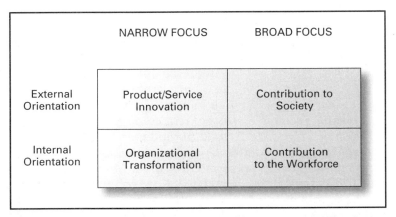

Figure 5–1 *A typology of visions. (Source: Conger, J. [1989]* The charismatic leader: Behind the mystique of exceptional leadership *[p. 44]. San
Francisco: Jossey-Bass.)*

to the patient." For example, a nursing unit might begin by developing or implementing critical pathways for a few classic diagnostic-related groups (DRGs). As this idea takes hold among nurses, physicians, and other healthcare providers, word about the positive patient outcomes and cost-effective results of using the critical paths would spread to the other departments in the organization (e.g., accounting, human resources, supplies, staffing). Consumer representatives who had served on the committees to institute the redesign would start sharing outcomes outside of the hospital, and soon there should be more external community and consumer interest.

WHY HAVE A VISION?

One can have personal and professional visions. Personal vision gives one a purpose in life, and professional vision helps one accomplish work ideas and the mission of the organization, group, or profession. One has to be able to identify when an opportunity presents to better the vision and act on incorporating whatever it is that would facilitate the implementation of the vision. One also has to be cognizant of the potential for "roadblocks" that are not going to aid in the vision becoming a reality. Plus, sometimes a roadblock may actually assist, in the long run, in mobilizing people to change and accept the new plan or vision.

For example, the advanced practice nurses (APNs) at a new inner-city nurse-run clinic felt "roadblocked" by their medical director, who insisted that all new prescription orders be cosigned by a physician before the medication could be dispensed. Concurrently, the clinic administrator was deliberating with the director of the adjacent detention center regarding servicing the inmates. One of the detention center's primary needs was immediate service, including prescriptions for a very transient, mobile clientele who might be at the jail for only 1 to 2 hours per day. A contract with the detention center would generate a large amount of work and a positive image for the clinic; however, no agreement could be made if the APNs could not independently get a medication dispensed. This roadblock of nurse practitioners not being able to autonomously prescribe new medications was finally overturned. The medical director was obliged to attend a meeting to discuss the role of the APNs and the state's APN practice act. This meeting would never have transpired if were not for the roadblocked prescriptions. The discussion resulted in several changes

> *"The secret of leadership is ... far-sightedness: gazing beyond the visible to the potential on the horizon."*
>
> —J. Donald Walters

that not only allowed the APNs to write new prescriptions but also expanded the scope of the APN and the mission of the nurse-run clinic even beyond the original vision.

ACTUALIZING A VISION

Many leaders have demonstrated the importance of being flexible, which is being able to accept some change in plans, to actualize a dream. When Bill Gates and Paul Allen founded Microsoft Corporation in 1975, their vision was to have a computer in every home, office, and school. Gates was only a college student at the time, but he was able to visualize a whole new role for computers in our personal lives. He took a leave from his undergraduate program at Harvard to follow his dream, and he took risks, used his creative talent, convinced others, and kept pursuing his dream. Today, Gates is in his early forties, and his company is the leading worldwide provider of personal computer (PC) software with revenues of $11 billion annually. If he had not left school when he did and risked going out on his own with Paul Allen, Bill Gates may have never actualized his dream and our world would not have been as dramatically changed by computers as we have witnessed in recent years. Such is the power of dreams—of visions (Manes & Andrews, 1993).

Mother Teresa, winner of a Nobel Peace Prize in 1979, founded the Missionaries of Charity in Calcutta, India. She had to make a difficult decision to leave the order of nuns to which she belonged at the time in order to follow her vision—"helping the poorest of the poor while living among them" (LeJoly, 1983, p. 26). Mother Teresa worked from morning to night helping the poor and guiding the nuns who joined her to fulfill her vision.

> *"Vision without action is merely a dream. Action without vision passes the time. Vision and action can change the world."*
> —Joel Baker

She was not satisfied with her purpose on earth as a nun in her original order, which was the status quo for her, so she took risks, used her creative talent, convinced others, and kept pursuing her dream, even without any funding. Mother Teresa founded a whole new order of sisters, provided exquisite care to the world's poor, and made the world more conscious of the needs of millions of our fellow human beings. Such is the power of dreams—of visions.

Kouzes and Posner (1993) describe leaders as pioneers—people who are able and willing to "reach for the sky," people who are able to recognize a great idea, and people who make change. Parse (1997) says a leader is "one who guides by blazing a path" (p. 109). She states that the path is a vision that offers something to others and that they can choose to follow or not. Many (Conger, 1989; Kotter, 1990; Porter-O'Grady & Wilson, 1995) believe that a leader's most significant function is to produce a change that cannot actually be identified as it transpires step by step but is more of a feeling that people grab onto, attempt to implement in their work, and then share serendipitously. Note that with the new leadership it would be nonproductive to be too orderly to attempt to implement a vision step by step, because ultimately no change would be generated. Porter-O'Grady and Wilson (1995) believe the pace of change in and the advancement of an organization or group are strongly correlated to the underlying vision that guides it. Although these authors hesitate to recommend short-term goal setting because they are proponents of the new science of leadership, they do advocate that managers become leaders and break down the barriers of the bureaucratic organizational structure of which we are all so much a part. Perhaps then, and only then, will leaders and followers be successful in owning a vision that is not in a locked-step goal format but rather leaves some possibilities for creative decision making.

Conger (1989) suggests that one positive advantage of having a vision is that it brings people a "sense of contribution to themselves, to an industry, or to a society." It also "draws workers together as a team" (p. 43). To share the same vision, followers must be inspired by the leader. Kotter (1990) suggests that leaders should stress the value of followers' contributions. Recognition for an extraordinary job in the form of an award, public announcement, or financial reimbursement might assist the follower to connect better to the overall vision.

An excellent example of a leader who had a dream, who motivated others, and who made followers feel as if they owned the dream was Dr. Martin Luther King, Jr. His "I Have a Dream" speech (Box 5–1), delivered on August 28, 1963, at the Lincoln Memorial in Washington, D.C., is a testament to the power of a vision and how it can energize people toward action.

Martin Luther King, Jr.'s, dream is clearly articulated, and the way he conveys his vision shows his passion and enthusiasm and the extent to which it comes from and reflects his inner being. Whether we work in administration, teaching, schools, homes, hospitals, or clinics—or whether we are students—each of us has a reason for why we became a nurse. That reason may have been to help others, to champion the "underdog," to care for others in need, or to develop healthcare programs for all. Perhaps some of us need to reflect on our original dream and think about how what we are currently doing relates to what we wanted to be nurses for

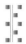

Box 5-1 *"I Have a Dream" by Martin Luther King, Jr.*

I say to you today, my friends, that in spite of the difficulties and frustrations of the moment I still have a dream. It is a dream deeply rooted in the American dream.

I have a dream that one day this nation will rise up and live out the true meaning of its creed: "We hold these truths to be self-evident, that all men are created equal."

I have a dream that one day on the red hills of Georgia the sons of former slaves and the sons of former slave owners will be able to sit down together at the table of brotherhood.

I have a dream that one day even the state of Mississippi, a desert state sweltering with the heat of injustice and oppression, will be transformed into an oasis of freedom and justice.

I have a dream that my four little children will one day live in a nation where they will not be judged by the color of their skin but by the content of their character.

I have a dream today.

I have a dream that one day the state of Alabama, whose governor's lips are presently dripping with the words of interposition and nullification, will be transformed into a situation where little black boys and black girls will be able to join hands with little white boys and white girls and walk together as sisters and brothers.

I have a dream today.

I have a dream that one day every valley shall be exalted, every hill and mountain shall be made low, the rough places will be made plains, and the crooked places will be made straight, and the glory of the Lord shall be revealed, and all flesh shall see it together.

This is our hope. This is the faith with which I return to the South. With this faith we will be able to transform the jangling discords of our nation into a beautiful symphony of brotherhood. With this faith we will be able to work together, to pray together, to struggle together, to go to jail together, to stand up for freedom together, knowing that we will be free one day.

(Continued)

Box 5–1   *"I Have a Dream" by Martin Luther King, Jr.—Concluded*

This will be the day when all of God's children will be able to sing with new meaning "My country 'tis of thee, sweet land of liberty, of thee I sing. Land where my fathers died, land of the pilgrim's pride, from every mountainside, let freedom ring."

And if America is to be a great nation this must become true. So let freedom ring from the prodigious hilltops of New Hampshire. Let freedom ring from the mighty mountains of New York. Let freedom ring from the heightening Alleghenies of Pennsylvania!

Let freedom ring from the snowcapped Rockies of Colorado!

Let freedom ring from the curvaceous peaks of California!

But not only that; let freedom ring from Stone Mountain of Georgia!

Let freedom ring from every hill and molehill of Mississippi. From every mountainside, let freedom ring!

When we let freedom ring, when we let it ring from every village and every hamlet, from every state and every city, we will be able to speed up that day when all of God's children, black men and white men, Jews and Gentiles, Protestants and Catholics, will be able to join hands and sing in the words of that old Negro spiritual, "Free at last! Free at last! Thank God almighty, we are free at last!"

Excerpt: Martin Luther King, Jr., speech delivered in Washington, D.C., on August 28, 1963. Source: Washington, J. (Ed.). (1992). *I have a dream: Writings and speeches that changed the world.* San Francisco: Harper.

in the first place. It is possible that our original idea of why we chose to enter nursing is still important and drives us to enjoy our present work; but it also is possible that we are stuck in a "dead end" or "rut" and feel that we are not fulfilled. We may get up day after day without thinking about why we do what we do. Perhaps it is time for a change, or maybe we need to revitalize ourselves.

By formulating a vision, we can take risks, use our creative talents, convince others, and keep pursuing our dreams. We can be energized and we can make a difference. We may have ideas about how the staffing mix could be more effective, how nurses could better collaborate with other members of the healthcare team, or how technology can be used better to improve patient outcomes. Any of these ideas could be the groundwork for our vision or our dream. Sometimes, an idea that starts out as one person's pet peeve or personal agenda—a computer in every home or school, helping the poorest of the poor, or achieving racial equality—can, if communicated effectively, become a group's quest. However one looks at it, one person's dream can excite others to follow or to envision their own separate piece of a larger vision. It seems that people who have dreams want to make a difference and are willing to do whatever it takes to fulfill those dreams. They believe that it is better to risk potential chaos than to accept the status quo. In other words, they are leaders in the fullest sense of the term.

Kouzes and Posner (1995, p. 120) suggest the following framework to use when developing a vision:

- Think first about your past.
- Determine what you want.
- Write an article about how you've made a difference.
- Write a short vision statement.
- Act on your intuition.
- Test your assumptions.
- Become a futurist.
- Rehearse with visualizations and affirmations.

For example, a nursing graduate student is applying for a scholarship. The application asks for the usual information about previous work, grade point average, memberships in professional organizations, and so forth and then requests applicants to share why they think they should be the winner of the scholarship. Using Kouzes and Posner's (1995) framework, the student could really make a case why he or she should be selected to receive this award: Describe your work as a staff nurse in terms of patient outcomes, creative teams you were a member or leader of, research you assisted with, protocols you helped develop; explain exactly why you are enrolled in your graduate program: specifically relate what you are doing in practice, what topics you are studying, and what issues you are researching; take this information and integrate it into how it is preparing you for your ideal job (your short vision statement); mention that you are in the process of submitting one of your papers as a manuscript for publication; share your gut feelings about healthcare, expand on one or two of your basic tenets of how you could really make a difference (use examples to maximize your viewpoints); and then conclude with your goals upon graduation and your expectations of yourself after 3 to 5 years. This vision possibly may snare that scholarship for the student, as well as serve as a professional guide for the individual to ascribe to during the next few years of working on his or her graduate degree.

WHAT HAPPENS IF THERE IS NO VISION?

When people wander aimlessly through their professional and personal lives, they tend not to accomplish the same results as someone who is a bit more focused (although open to change). They may not take advantage of an opportunity for professional growth because they were unaware of it even happening, or in terms of a personal aspect of their life, they may be unable to go on the "vacation of a lifetime" because they have a conflicting business engagement already scheduled. Manfredi (1995) described the art of legendary leadership with the following story, which depicts what can happen if there is no vision: Many years ago the long-term mayor of a village passed away. The town elders gathered to select a successor. They asked for volunteers and after awhile three candidates were found. There were no job description or selection criteria. The elders decided to test the candidates' leadership by placing each in charge of the village for one month. Whoever was most successful would become the mayor. #1 Candidate believed he should keep the village stable and his motto became: "No need to grow, support the status quo." #2 Candidate believed one must create structure in order to lead and so he developed many rules and regulations. He felt rules were made only for subjects and not leaders. So the elders had a bonfire and burned all 700 volumes of rules that had been developed. #3 Candidate felt leaders know what is best for the general public and that villagers cannot be trusted to make decisions or develop ideas. So for one month he made all of the decisions and never consulted them. After one month the elders made a decision to get rid of him. All three candidates were rejected. The elders could not come to an agreement as to exactly what the role of a leader should be so they went off and discussed this for awhile. They finally came up with five roles for a leader to possess: "Leaders create visions, leaders create climates, leaders create conflict, leaders create change, and leaders create leaders" (p. 62).

Basically, if a person does not have a vision, he or she cannot create a climate for conflict, change, and growth. Without conflict, change, and growth, new leaders will not be able to emerge from a group to inspire further conflict, change, and growth, and therefore the status quo is perpetuated by the "leader who knows best for the group" by adhering to the "same old, same old" rules and regulations.

WHO SHOULD PARTICIPATE IN VISION DEVELOPMENT?

Bennis (1989) believes that one can learn how to develop a vision. Manfredi (1995) makes the point that anyone, not only the leader, can initiate an idea, which is visionary. It is the idea that sparks the vision, which is the most significant part of developing a vision; and we all have had creative ideas that others have been most interested in hearing about. Sometimes an individual will come up with a thought and then someone else will add to it and then another person will expand it even more. Soon the entire group of people will be involved in the idea, and a change in practice will be generated. This process can be applied perhaps to developing a more global change in staffing, a philosophy of patient care, or a new nursing-driven protocol, which, in the past, may have been dependent on a physician. Take, for example, staff nurses discussing the disadvantages of caring for intravenous lines of patients with hard-to-stick veins. One nurse says how difficult she finds it having to insert a new line just about every 4 hours and having to hurt the patient and explain why it is necessary to the patient and the family over and over again. Another nurse suggests that it is time for nurses to select appropriate patients for routine intravenous access or for a more invasive line and for nurses to insert the peripherally inserted central catheter (PICC) and manage the patients who have these more invasive lines. This idea of providing the nurse with more independence regarding intravenous fluid and medication administration could easily just be the starting point for an even bigger dream—the independence to have significantly more nurse-driven protocols so that higher-quality care, as well as more cost-effective care, could be generated. In nursing, it usually is the direct care provider nurses who are most aware of what is best for the client and ultimately what would improve the way care is delivered. Such nurses have ideas, dreams, and visions. Sadly, however, they often fail to do anything significant about them. Although it generally falls to the leader to actually implement a vision, everyone in the group needs to be involved to achieve success.

In a classic article on leaders and vision, Zaleznik (1989) suggests two ways to persuade people: (1) make sure they realize that certain actions will assist their interests, and (2) attempt to change the way they value their motives. Both the leader and the followers, therefore, need to be immersed in the process of acquiring the vision and integrating it into their everyday operation. The vision leader also needs to be available for followers as they need assistance in clarifying the vision, seeing how their efforts contribute to the vision, and being passionate about working toward the vision.

STRATEGIES TO ASSIST PEOPLE WITH VISION DEVELOPMENT

Having positive experience with trying new things, being involved in new opportunities, and being encouraged to be entrepreneurial will assist anyone in succeeding with vision development. In 1991 Sarah Weddington, past counsel for *Roe v. Wade,* delivered a keynote speech at the National League for Nursing Annual Convention in which she shared several ideas on how to gain practice in leading. The major focus of her presentation was that a leader must be passionate about what he or she does and must always strive to accomplish his or her dream. The dream must be a product of what would be the ideal and what would have the most positive impact for the future. So, a successful vision not only needs to encompass many details and perspectives but also must include some bearing on how the vision will affect the future. The idea is to follow Sarah Weddington's advice that people must be proactive and not shy away from new things. Rather, take time to try a different way, think about something in a whole new fashion, and have the confidence from past experience of engaging in new experiences to encourage others to come along and share the dream.

> *"Harry Truman was right, it's the leaders who shape history. There would have been no United States without Thomas Jefferson, no Third Reich without Adolph Hitler. But no man or woman becomes a leader unless he or she wants to. They've got to have a burning need to get there."*
>
> —Robert Ludlum (in *The Icarus Agenda*, p. 264)

One can learn how to communicate a vision in an articulate and persuasive manner. Conger (1989) suggests that the leader use metaphors and analogies to excite others and that the leader stimulate multiple senses (intellect, emotions, values, and imagination) simultaneously. Abraham Lincoln used great emphasis in his conclusion of the Gettysburg Address when he said: "government of the people, for the people, and by the people" instead of saying "government of, for, and by the people" (Conger, 1989, p. 169). Franklin Delano Roosevelt tended to use folk imagery to share his ideas with the citizenry and he used sports analogies in his fireside chats (Conger, 1989, p. 81); both were things with which people could easily relate. Another example of someone who related well at the grassroots level and established trust was Lee Iacocca, former CEO of Chrysler. Iacocca expressed his dream to rebuild the car company and his willingness to give everything it would take when he announced that he would accept a $1.00 salary for the whole year. Such a strategy created a strong identification between Iacocca and the average Chrysler employee, and it demonstrated an extraordinary level of personal commitment to a vision (Conger, 1989, pp. 73–74).

Although some leaders may be inclined to try to convince others with impressive numbers, Conger (1989) asserts that statistical summaries are uninformative and lack impact because they are colorless. He suggests "brief face-to-face comments" as being most substantial in getting people to buy into an idea or make a change (p. 76). Other speech techniques such as repetition, rhythm, and alliteration are effective in helping articulate one's vision, as is evident in Martin Luther King, Jr.'s "I Have a Dream" speech. Conger also suggests that one use a loud volume, some body movements, and complete sentences with few pauses between them. It also is helpful to avoid "I think," "I guess," "please," and "thank you" and just stick to the basic message so that the speaker is portrayed as confident, effective, and someone others would want to follow. Leaders must be able to communicate their vision effectively, a skill that many believe is the most important characteristic of being a leader (Bennis & Nanus, 1985; Nanus, 1992).

Nurses in practice today are knowledgeable and sophisticated. Therefore the leader must be able to communicate a very well-thought-out vision, but at the same time a vision that can be changed to incorporate the team's ideas. A framework of skills is needed to be successful in articulating, communicating, and propelling a vision. Senge (1994) says a leader of healthcare must be a systems thinker, have shared visioning, facilitate team learning, and have personal mastery.

> *"Look before you leap ... or you'll find yourself behind."*
> —Benjamin Franklin

Champy (1995) agrees with his list of competencies for healthcare leaders, including association, collaboration, communication, and mobilizing skills. Drucker (1989) reaffirms these similar lists with his: coaching, knowledge of technology, visionary, and facilitator skills. All three of these organizational behaviorists agree on the necessity of a leader being able to communicate the dream—this is the main point for our existence.

To sum up all of these ideas about vision, think of a sailor who must return to port in the middle of a thunderstorm with barely 3 feet of visibility. The best thing the sailor can do is concentrate on the ultimate destination, not on every foot of sea between him and land. This metaphor can be used in describing the journey a group, organization, or professional takes in reaching the dream. One must constantly look forward even if it takes a long time, lots of work, and energy expenditure to get there. To "keep on track," the leader must help all members of the group feel a sense of ownership and must be creative throughout the process of moving toward a vision.

The Process of Creativity

The essence of creativity is "not the possession of some special talent, it is much more the ability to play" (Bennis, 1989, p. 95). Creativity "demands intuition, uncertainty, unconventionality, and individual expression" (Conger, 1989, p. 17). Creativity, as it relates to leaders, occurs when leaders transform their experiences into ideas (Valiga & Bruderle, 1997). Leadership is about "creating a new way of life" and changing the "business as usual environment" (Kouzes & Posner, 1993, pp. 37–39). If chaos is the reality of the 1990s, as many experts claim, creativity is one skill we will need to appreciate, develop, and incorporate to successfully navigate this white-water turbulence.

Creativity involves believing that "there is no one answer that is right but many answers that might work" (Wheatley & Kellner-Rogers, 1996, p. 16). As nurses we must reframe how we think about our jobs to be more creative, more open to a variety of possibilities, and more open to options that might work. Perhaps we will need to become more involved in developing programs for outpatients to attend, writing grants to obtain funding for health promotion programs, educating patients on a larger scope, trying different staff mix patterns to best meet patient needs, being more flexible with time schedules to include 9- or 7-hour shifts depending on unit needs, developing healthcare policies, serving on political action boards as a representative for health promotion affairs, and any number of other activities that will improve healthcare for people. In other words, nurses will have to become more comfortable with ambiguity and uncertainty so that they can see "new forms take shape, new ideas develop, and new goals fulfilled" (Valiga & Bruderle, 1997, p. 234). Most probably, it is easier to increase creativity by changing conditions in the work setting or home atmo-sphere than by influencing people to think in a more creative fashion (Csikszentmihalyl, 1996). In other words, it may be easier to focus on providing a creative ambiance in schools, day-care centers, homes, churches, and work settings than actually trying to make a person think more creatively without influencing the environment.

"Leaders invent themselves" and they are "not born, but made, . . . usually self-made"(Bennis, 1989, pp. 45–46). Leaders are curious and daring. They "embrace errors, knowing they will learn from them" (p. 39). Leaders shape life, rather than just being shaped by it (p. 79). All of these statements has relevance for the individual nurse who is a leader or an effective follower. It is no longer acceptable for nurses to deal only with the here and now of a specific patient assignment in the hospital or home setting. Nurse leaders should partner with the patient and form alliances with family members, community groups, and other healthcare professionals to provide needed health teaching, promote self-competence for the patient, and gather relevant data to determine whether desired outcomes are being realized. It is time to change our belief that what we have known is all there is, and it is time to change our belief that how things are done has to be the way things continue to be done. Wheatley and Kellner-Rogers (1996, pp. 13–14) challenge us with the following beliefs about life creating itself:

Everything is in a constant process of discovery and creating. Everything is changing all of the time: individuals, systems, environments, the rules, and the processes of evolution. Even change changes. Every organism reinterprets the rules, creates exceptions for itself, creates new rules.

Life uses messes to get to well-ordered solutions. Life doesn't seem to share our desires for efficiency or neatness. It uses redundancy, fuzziness, dense webs of relationships, and unending trials and errors to find what works.

Life is intent on finding what works, not what's right. It is the ability to keep finding solutions that is important; any one solution is temporary. There are no permanently right answers. The capacity to keep changing, to find what works now, is what keeps any organism alive.

Life creates more possibilities as it engages with opportunities. There are no "windows of opportunity," narrow openings in the fabric of space-time that soon disappear forever. Possibilities beget more possibilities; they are infinite.

Life is attracted to order. It experiments until it discovers how to form a system that can support diverse members. Individuals search out a wide range of possible relationships to discover whether they can organize into a life-sustaining system. These explorations continue until a system is discovered. This system then provides stability for its members, so that individuals are less buffeted by change.

Life organizes around identity. Every living thing acts to develop and preserve itself. Identity is the filter that every organism or system uses to make sense of the world. New information, new relationships, changing environments—all are interpreted through a sense of self. This tendency toward self-creation is so strong that it creates a seeming paradox. An organism will change to maintain its identity.

Everything participates in the creation and evolution of its neighbors. There are no unaffected outsiders. No one system dictates conditions to another. All participate together in creating the conditions of their interdependence.

Obviously, there is no one right answer, there is no way anyone can plan for all of the potential problems that might occur when attempting to institute creative and innovative approaches to reach a vision, and there is no room for a "getting everything right" attitude because everything will continue to change and some sort of acceptable order will emerge. Perhaps as nurses we should develop our right brain skills more so that we can be more intuitive, conceptual, and artistic instead of being dominated by the left side of the brain with our logical planning, to-do lists, and conservative perspective. Bennis (1989) suggests we be whole brained so that both concrete and abstract ideas can be used. For example, the Mindmap of Creativity (Fig. 5–2) depicts various actions that a creative person uses. Mindmapping is a method of note taking that could be effective in stimulating our creativity and developing our right-brain skills. Approaches like this can stimulate the flow of ideas from our more concrete left brain. This exercise of illustrating what one reads or sees may be a helpful exercise in developing the whole brain.

Think back to when you were in first grade. How do you think your teacher would have reacted if you gave an answer such as the one shown in Fig. 5–3? For most of us, the teacher probably would have scolded us for being too right-brained! Educators, nurse educators in particular, can assist the profession by designing learning experiences that allow for student creativity and the use of skills governed by both the right and left sides of the brain. In this way, nursing will not consist of all task-oriented left-brain thinkers or all right-brain thinkers.

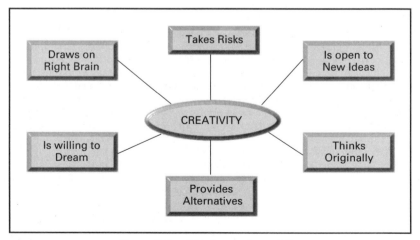

Figure 5–2 *Mindmap of creativity.*

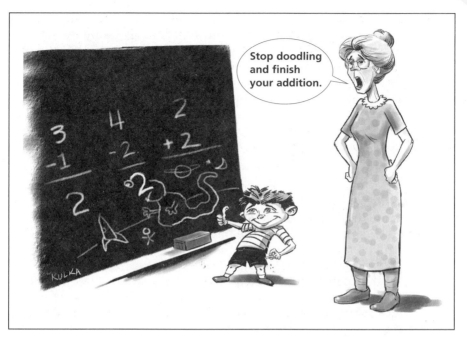

Figure 5–3 *Using our right brain.*

Nurses also must focus less energy on and worry less about some unknown future; instead we should focus more on the opportunities before us today and the possibilities awaiting us tomorrow. Thinking more openly, being more aware of possibilities, and being less structured and more creative will take us a long way. "If we believe that the world is self-organizing, then we don't have to be the organizers; in fact, we don't have to struggle to create networks, affiliations, or teams, . . . groups will just happen" (Wheatley & Kellner-Rogers, 1996, p. 35).

So in healthcare today, the mergers, acquisitions, affiliations, and partnering are really not a bad thing but a natural force; a bringing together of talent, resources, and one hopes, better patient outcomes. Our ability to be creative and use the networking will ultimately allow us to survive. We must foster rethinking, discovery, and curiosity and support the changes. This is the new way of thinking about leadership, and we have to change our way of thinking about our responsibilities. "In a self-organizing system, people do for themselves most of what in the past has been done to them. Self-organizing systems create their own structures, patterns of behavior, and processes for accomplishing their work. They design what is necessary to do the work. They agree on behaviors and relationships that make sense to them. Those of us

irectly involved in the doing of their work can give up fussing
ut designs, or believing that our timelines make things hap-
, or that our training programs change the behavior of the or-
nization" (Wheatley & Kellner-Rogers, 1996, p. 38). We can
support one another, trust one another, and create possibilities or
dreams never thought of before, if we can just balance out our
need to organize every tiny detail and, instead, allow ourselves to
be creative. "Basically getting people to reach beyond their best
abilities is knowing how to manage creativity" (Sculley, 1987).

THE SIGNIFICANCE OF CREATIVITY

Creativity is necessary if nurses are to have a positive view of the
multitude of changes occurring in healthcare today and that are expected to continue well into the future. "Downsizing," "merging,"
and "affiliating" are buzzwords that to most nurses mean a change
in responsibilities or a loss of job. If nurses could muster some
entrepreneurialism, we could undergo some serious growth as a
profession and as individuals despite downsizing, mergers, and acquisitions. Porter-O'Grady (1997) describes how he has succeeded in
the role of a consultant and entrepreneur. He shares that the secret of
his career has been good mentors, seizing the opportunity to try
something new even when he was not sure he was prepared for it,
and accepting changes in his professional and personal life. His rec-
ommendation to fellow nurses is to gather practice and skills in facilitation, creativity, leadership, and design (p. 29).

Being able to try new things, challenge traditional ways of thinking and behaving, and be open to new ways of thinking can only
broaden our visions. We cannot let ourselves accept that all "flowers
are red [and] green leaves are green" (Chapin, 1978). The words to
Harry Chapin's song "Flowers Are Red," for example, illustrate what
can happen when individuals are not allowed to think creatively.
Creativity is what will allow us to accomplish our visions with excitement and enthusiasm. One gets a resurgence of energy when something new and exciting occurs or when one has an "a-ha" insight.
But this energy also comes from change itself, and when that change
relates to our work and what we do, we can experience phenomenal
growth. "Work comes from the inside out, work is an expression of
our soul, our inner being. It's unique to the individual, it's creative"
(Fox, 1994, p. 49). Work, therefore, should not be boring, repetitious,
tiring, and frustrating. Instead, it should be and can be energizing,
challenging, rewarding, and growth-producing.

USING CREATIVITY

Nurses should be using their creative strategies to staff units, research new protocols, administer medications and treatments,

communicate patient information to other professionals, develop materials to market nurses' skills for patients at home, plan support groups for inpatients and outpatients, or build partnerships with a clinic or a school-based healthcare provider. For too long, nurses have been accustomed to staying in the same environment (home, long-term care facility, school, clinic, or hospital) for an entire career. But as new roles emerge and new settings provide opportunities for nurses, there is no need to feel stuck or to be stuck. Nurses are becoming more directly patient-oriented and more independent, practicing autonomously and in multiple environments. Today, nurses are expected to be vital members of multidisciplinary health team efforts, they are willing to do things differently, they revise protocols to be more patient-oriented, they focus on measuring patient outcomes, and they are concerned about providing quality, cost-effective care.

McCall (1989) suggests some interesting methods by which leaders can use creative strategies to clarify and achieve their visions. By being "feisty," leaders can deliberately create conflicts to spark new ideas between selected, key people and propel their ideas forward. Creative leaders also are "crafty" in that they are politically astute, they know how to increase their power base, and they can enlist broad support for some creative, different pursuit. If creative leaders are to survive, they must be able to disassociate with failure and associate with success. Being creative puts a leader in a bit of danger because it involves taking risks. A sense of "grouchiness" also is generally necessary for a creative leader because one would have to be very demanding to help everyone involved with the new idea to meet the highest, most impeccable standards. Another interesting strategy is pushing everyone to their utmost to work their hardest and be highly motivated employees. McCall (1989) goes so far as to say that a creative leader has to act before thinking rather than think before acting and has to be inconsistent so that the leader can keep the system "open" for new ideas and changes. Last, creative leaders must use intuition and hunches so that they do not miss a potentially new way to accomplish the vision. By using these strategies in any nursing role, it would be difficult to become bored with a job, to burn out, or to feel stuck.

CONCLUSION

There is no doubt that leaders must be passionate about their visions, their dreams of making significant differences or bettering the world. It is also crucial that leaders be able to persuade people to "grab on" to this vision and become involved in creating the change. As Zaleznik (1989) noted, one cannot be successful without using one's imagination and being more comfortable with disorder and chaos. In other words, we need to avoid the "If it ain't broke, don't fix it" way of thinking (p. 62). Change will occur no matter what we do to maintain the existing order. If we have articulated worthy visions, if we have discovered the notion of creativity, and if we use creative strategies to achieve our vision, we will thrive on this change, grow personally, and be effective leaders who shape a better world.

"Vision is the art of seeing things invisible."

—Jonathan Swift

Critical Thinking Exercises

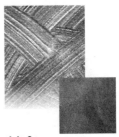

Read the story "Footprints." How does this relate to creativity? to leadership? to providing leadership and fostering creativity in nursing?

"Footprints"

In a faraway land long ago, there was once a wise and good village chief who had a most exciting announcement. "Of utmost importance," he reminded his villagers, "is the ability to travel to the port to trade our jewelry for food. Until recently those traveling to the port simply left our village and wandered aimlessly until they either found the port or died. I am happy to announce that thanks to the efforts of our wise and most scientific medicine man we have captured the essence of travel. We have discovered that all travel is based on footprints. Follow footprints precisely and you will never get lost going to or from the port again."

"But what about trees?" asked one villager.

"Trees are not footprints, and trees should be ignored," replied the chief.

"May we consider the stars?" questioned another.

"Don't be foolish," commanded the chief. "What could be farther from footprints than stars? Have I not told you already? There is no travel without footprints. Footprints are the essence of travel. Understand footprints, and the concept of travel is yours forever. You will never be lost again."

That was many years ago. And since that time many villagers have come and gone from the port, never taking their eyes off the footprints. Some of the more scholarly villagers over the years have studied and refined footprintology, writing long, scholarly discourses on the many things that footprints show, and of the many truths to be found through scrutiny of footprints.

Over the years the methods of observing footprints have been refined to such an exact science that many years of studying with rigorous examinations are required to truly practice and teach footprintology. In fact, before each young man is able to leave the village he must be thoroughly educated in footprintology as the essence of travel, lest some day he look up at the trees or stars and lose sight of that essence that the wisest of wise know as travel.

Source: Bagley, D. (1979). Footprints (a parable about knowledge). *Journal of Creative Behavior, 13* (4), 286–287.

_____

_____

What is your vision for nursing in general? in your current sphere of practice? What goals do you have for the profession? Which of these goals can be achieved by nurses themselves, and which need external "approval" or action?

_____

_____

Using Martin Luther King, Jr.'s "I Have A Dream" speech (see Box 5–1) or the speeches of other powerful orators (e.g., John F. Kennedy, Margaret Thatcher, Abraham Lincoln), identify communication methods you could use to articulate your dream clearly.

_____

_____

Compare and contrast an experience you've had professionally to Harry Chapin's song "Flowers Are Red." How could you use "every color" to prevent a recurrence?

_____

_____

Create a mindmap of leadership.

_____

_____

Complete the "How Creative Are You?" questionnaire. What did you learn about yourself?

_____

_____

How Creative Are You?

Directions. Below are 30 statements that are useful in determining a person's current level of creativity. Read each statement. Answer "A" for those statements with which you "Agree" Answer "B" for those statements on which you are "In Between" or "Don't Know." Answer "C" for those with which you DISAGREE.

1. I always work with a great deal of certainty that I'm following the correct procedures for solving a particular problem. _____

2. It would be a waste of time for me to ask questions if I had no hope of obtaining answers. _____

3. I concentrate harder on whatever interests me than do most people. _____

4. I feel that a logical step-by-step method is best for solving problems. _____

5. I occasionally voice opinions in groups that seem to turn people off. _____

6. It is more important for me to do what I believe to be right than to try to win the approval of others. _____

7. More than other people, I need to have things interesting and exciting. _____

8. I am able to stick with difficult problems over extended periods of time. _____

9. On occasion I get overly enthusiastic about things. _____

10. I often get my best ideas when doing nothing in particular. _____

11. I rely on intuitive hunches and the feeling of "rightness" or "wrongness" when moving toward the solution of a problem. _____

12. I like hobbies that involve collecting things. _____

13. Daydreaming has provided the impetus for many of my more important projects. _____

14. I have a high degree of aesthetic sensitivity. _____

15. I am driven to achieve positions or situations of power in life. _____

16. I like people who are most sure of their conclusions. _____

17. Inspiration has nothing to do with successful solution of problems. _____

18. I am much more interested in coming up with new ideas than I am trying to sell them to others. _____

19. I would enjoy spending an entire day alone, just "chewing the mental cud." _____

20. I tend to avoid situations in which I might feel inferior. _____

21. I resent things being uncertain and unpredictable. _____

22. I like people who follow the rule, "business before pleasure." _____

23. Self-respect is much more important than the respect of others. _____

24. I feel that people who strive for perfection are unwise. _____

25. I prefer to work with others in a team effort rather than solo. _____

26. I like work in which I must influence others. _____

27. Many problems that I encounter in life cannot be resolved in terms of right or wrong solutions. _____

28. It is important for me to have a place for everything, everything in its place. _____

29. I prefer writers who write so that the average person can understand them to those who use strange or fancy words. _____

30. I would be more comfortable in a job that had a steady routine than I would in a job in which a person would have to do different things every day. _____

After having selected an "A," "B," or "C" response to each statement, follow the scoring in-structions to determine your current level of creativity. To compute your score, circle your response to each statement and add up the value assigned to each item.

Statement Number	A	B	C
1.	0	1	2
2.	0	1	2
3.	4	1	2
4.	−2	0	3
5.	2	1	0
6.	3	0	−1
7.	3	0	−1
8.	4	1	0
9.	3	0	−1
10.	2	1	0
11.	4	0	−2
12.	0	1	2
13.	3	0	−1
14.	3	0	−1
15.	0	1	2
16.	−1	0	2
17.	0	1	3
18.	2	1	0
19.	2	0	−1
20.	0	1	2
21.	0	1	2
22.	0	1	2
23.	3	0	—
24.	−1	0	2
25.	0	1	2
26.	1	2	2
27.	2	1	0
28.	0	1	2
29.	−1	0	2
30.	−1	1	3

65–75 = Exceptionally creative   16–29 = Average
49–64 = Very creative   8–15 = Below average
30–48 = Above average   15–7 = Uncreative

Source: Raudsepp, E. (1981). *How creative are you?* New York: Putnam.

References

Bagley, D. (1979). Footprints (a parable about knowledge). *Journal of Creative Behavior 13*(4), 286–287.

Bennis, W. (1989). *On becoming a leader.* Reading, MA: Addison-Wesley.

Bennis, W., & Nanus, B. (1985). *Leaders: The strategies for taking charge.* New York: Harper & Row.

Champy, J. (1995). *Reengineering management.* New York: HarperBusiness.

Chapin, H. (1978). Flowers are red. *Legends of the lost and found album.* New York: Electra/Asylum Records, Division of Warner Communications, Inc.

Conger, J. (1989). *The charismatic leader: Behind the mystique of exceptional leadership.* San Francisco: Jossey-Bass.

Csikszentmihalyl, M. (1996). *Creativity flow and the psychology of discovery and intervention.* New York: HarperCollins.

Drucker, P. (1989). *The new realities.* New York: Harper & Row.

Fox, M. (1994). *Reinvention of work: A new vision of livelihood for our time.* San Francisco: Harper.

Kotter, J. (1990). *A force for change.* New York: The Free Press.

Kouzes, J., & Posner, B. (1995). *The leadership challenge.* San Francisco: Jossey-Bass.

Kouzes, J., & Posner, B. (1993). *Credibility.* San Francisco: Jossey-Bass.

LeJoly, E. (1983). *Mother Teresa of Calcutta.* New York: Harper & Row.

Manes, S., & Andrews, P. (1993). *Gates: How Microsoft's mogul reinvented an industry and made himself the richest man in America.* New York: Doubleday.

Manfredi, C. (1995). The art of legendary leadership: lessons for new and aspiring leaders. *Nursing Leadership Forum 1*(2), 62–64.

McCall, M. (1989). Conjecturing about creative leaders. In W.E. Rosenbach & R.L. Taylor (Eds.), *Contemporary issues in leadership* (2ⁿᵈ ed.) (pp. 111–120). Boulder, CO: Westveiw Press.

Nanus, B. (1992). *Visionary leadership.* San Francisco: Jossey-Bass.

Parse, R. (1997). Leadership: The essentials. *Nursing Science Quarterly 10*(3), 109.

Porter-O'Grady, T. (1997). The private practice of nursing: The gift of entrepreneurialism. *Nursing Administration Quarterly 22*(1), 23–29.

Porter-O'Grady, T., & Wilson, C. (1995). *The leadership revolution in health care: Altering systems, changing behaviors.* Gaithersburg, MD: Aspen.

Raudsepp, E. (1981). *How creative are you?* New York: Putnam.

Sashkin, M. (1989). Visionary leadership: A perspective from education. In W.E. Rosenbach & R.L. Taylor (Eds.), *Contemporary issues in leadership* (2ⁿᵈ ed.) (pp. 222–234). Boulder, CO: Westview Press.

Sculley, J. (1987). Sculley's lessons from inside Apple. *Fortune,* September 14, 1987, *116,* 108–111.

Senge, P. (1994). *The fifth discipline.* New York: Doubleday Currency.

Valiga, T., & Bruderle, E. (1997). *Using the arts and humanities to teach nursing: A creative approach.* New York: Springer.

Washington, J. (Ed.). (1992). *I have a dream: Writings and speeches that changed the world.* San Francisco: Harper.

Wheatley, M., & Kellner-Rogers, M. (1996). *A simpler way.* San Francisco: Berrett-Koehler.

Zaleznik, A. (1989). Why managers lack vision. *Business Month*, August, 59–64.

CHAPTER 6

Gender Perspectives in Leadership

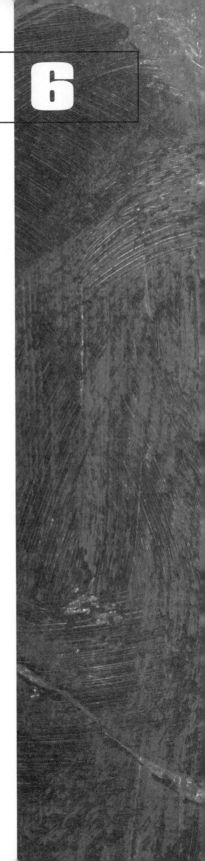

Gender Perspectives in Leadership

Learning Objectives

☐ Compare "feminine leadership" with "masculine leadership."

☐ Examine the concept of androgyny.

☐ Describe barriers women face to exercising leadership in organizations.

☐ Propose strategies that women and men can use to enhance their effectiveness as leaders in organizations.

☐ Compare "web" organizations with "hierarchical" ones.

INTRODUCTION

As has been noted, most of the studies that have been done about leaders and leadership have focused on men and the male perspective. Although this information is valuable and much of what we know about leadership—the need to have a vision, the reciprocal relationship between leaders and followers, the willingness to take risks, and so on—has broad applicability, it still is rooted largely in a "masculine" framework. There is a growing body of literature, however, that notes differences in the ways women lead (Felder, 1996; Gordon, 1991; Grunwald, 1992; Helgesen, 1990a; Kram & Hampton, 1998; Lipman-Blumen, 1992; Long, 1998; Melia & Lyttle, 1986; Rosener, 1990; Schein, 1989). Because most nurses are women, understanding gender perspectives in leadership is an essential area of exploration.

This chapter explores some of the "typical stereotypes" about differences between men and women and how they translate into (1) differences in each gender's approach to leadership and (2) different types of organizational structures that best "fit" with each approach. This chapter also examines ways in which the best of both worlds can be combined into a truly effective leader.

Common Gender Differences

Leaders reflect the values, norms, strengths, and weaknesses of their groups and, indeed, of the larger society. Although this usually is considered a strength and an advantage, it can present a challenge for the leader who is a woman and who is functioning in "a man's world."

"Maleness" often is associated with ideas such as dominance, independence, objectivity, rationality, competitiveness, aggressiveness, boldness, decisiveness, toughness, being logical, and being "thing-oriented." These are terms that also are often associated with leadership, and masculine traits, therefore, often are equated with effective leadership skills (Stivers, 1991). "Femaleness," on the other hand, typically is associated with ideas that are not aligned with leadership, ideas such as compliance, dependence, emotionality, weakness, being accepting, passivity, nurturance, and being "people-oriented." Comparisons such as those noted in Table 6–1 often are made in jest, but the basis of them is all too real for women in many arenas.

| Table 6-1 | *A Businessman versus a Businesswoman* |

Businessman	**Businesswoman**
A businessman is aggressive.	A businesswoman is pushy.
A well-dressed businessman is fashionable.	A well-dressed businesswomen is a "clotheshorse."
He loses his temper because he's so involved with his job.	She's "bitchy."
He's a man of the world.	She's "been around."
He's confident.	She's conceited.
He drinks because of excessive work pressures.	She's a lush.
He's enthusiastic.	She's emotional.
He's careful about details.	She's picky.
He's depressed (or hung over), so everyone tiptoes past his office.	She's moody, so it must be "her time of the month."
He follows through.	She doesn't know when to quit.
He's firm.	She's stubborn.
He makes wise judgments.	She reveals her prejudices.
He isn't afraid to say what he thinks.	She's opinionated.
He exercises authority.	She's tyrannical.
He's discreet.	She's secretive.
He's a stern taskmaster.	She's difficult to work for.

Although it is no longer remarkable to find women in positions of authority, power, and leadership, most women in the workforce still are clustered at the bottom of the employment "heap" (e.g., clerical jobs, low-paying professional jobs). It also has been shown that most individuals with political influence are men, and organizational heads tend not to be women. One report (Brooks, 1983) noted that "rather than being trained for the new technologies, many [women] wind up being taught only to master a few specific data-processing tasks that cannot be easily transferred" (p. 31). Therefore they are limited in what they can do, the opportunities they can pursue, and the breadth or possibly even the significance of contributions they can make to an organization. Ultimately their opportunities for advancement, personal growth, and leadership are limited.

Reasons why there are a limited number of women exercising leadership are many, including the following: society does not expect and value leadership in women, women typically are not socialized as leaders, there are few women leader role models, and women who do try to exert strong leadership behaviors sometimes are discriminated against and not supported in those efforts. It also has been claimed that women fear success and that they are fearful of competition. In addition, it is common to see references to the "Queen Bee syndrome," in which women "at the top" want to be only with men, want to keep other women down, and downplay the concerns expressed by women who are trying to succeed with comments such as, "I did it without much help. Why can't you?"

Many women, however, have challenged the "system," overcome these fears, dealt with the "Queen Bees," and obtained the education, training, and skills needed to compete effectively and move into positions of power and leadership. As a result, these hard-working, ambitious women may be seen as a threat to men and other women. Therefore they need to invest energies into dealing with all the stereotype issues (e.g., being perceived as threats, not being "real" women), as well as dealing with the issues inherent in the job itself (e.g., improving the bottom line, producing a product before the competition does).

The challenges that women face in pursuing leadership roles clearly are related to early socialization. Assumptions are made about what is appropriate for girls and boys (e.g., "boys don't cry or play with dolls," and "girls are emotional and prefer more isolated play activities rather than competitive team sports"). Relationships develop based on these assumptions, they become deeply ingrained over time through experiences such as school (American Association of University Women, 1992), and socialization along these lines continues throughout adulthood. It is the woman, for example, who is more likely to have to struggle to balance work, family responsibilities, and other commitments because our society—even though changes continue to be made toward greater sharing of responsibilities—continues to allow the male partner to emphasize the work or professional role while expecting the female partner to "do it all."

Women who attempt to break away from these stereotypes often are regarded as "deviant" (Vance, 1979). Deviance is thought to occur when an individual varies too widely from the norm and fails to obey group rules. It is considered essentially pathological and a symptom of social disorganization. Thus women who assert themselves as leaders may be viewed negatively by the larger society.

Even women who do achieve high positions may be viewed with less credibility and respect than their male counterparts, and they may be criticized by male and female peers alike. Woman leaders also may be considered inferior and "second class." Despite these challenges, however, women bring a unique dimension to leadership roles.

Women's Ways of Leading

Although distinctions between men and women often are outlined in a humorous way (as noted in Table 6–1), differences between their styles and the way they lead have been reported. For example, the "Alpha" and "Beta" types of leadership described by Levenstein (1981) may be aligned with masculine and feminine leadership. According to this author, Alpha leadership is analytic, relies heavily on rationale, is quantitative, relies on hierarchical relationships, and favors engineered solutions; it is a style that thrives on competitive challenges and sees power as a goal. In comparison, Beta leadership is intuitive, qualitative, and concerned about growth; it relies on support relationships and is future-oriented. It is a style in which power is seen as a means to a goal that has relevance for the members of the group and those served by the group, rather than a goal in and of itself or a means to a goal that has relevance only for the leader. Alpha leadership might be more closely aligned with a male perspective, and Beta leadership might be more reflective of female leadership.

> *"Women tend to stick it out too long and just try to work harder for recognition."*
> —Marie Wunsch

These kinds of differences in thinking and leadership styles can have significant ramifications, as was pointed out in a brief piece related to military force (Sexes Differ on Military Force, 1985). This piece noted that having more women in the House and Senate could significantly alter decision making in the American political arena. It reported on the work of two Canadian researchers who concluded that women were less likely than men to support funding for nuclear weapons and missile testing and more likely to favor deterrence through disarmament rather than

Cold War. Men, these researchers noted, tended to be not only more "pro-force" than women but also tended to see military defense issues in more "simplistic terms." Women tended to view the same issues from a more complex, "holistic" perspective that included the "human dimension." The researchers concluded that men and women organized their thoughts differently: "If nothing else, males had a much simpler perspective on things and tended to see issues in black and white terms . . . but women saw shades of gray" (Sexes differ on military force, 1985, p. 7). Cold War issues are no longer of major concern in our society, as they were in 1985 when this report was issued. Nevertheless, the findings of this study regarding women's perspectives, their tendency to be more nurturing and "other-oriented," the priorities that play into their decision making, and the ways in which their thinking and potential leadership differ from men are worth noting.

> *"Transformational leadership feels right to women because it's not asking anything that they haven't done."*
>
> —Jacquelyn M. Belcher

Rosener (1990) described four major areas of difference in style exhibited by the women leaders she studied: they tended to encourage participation, they shared power and information quite readily, they were concerned about enhancing the self-worth of others, and they worked to energize others. This is consistent with other descriptions of women leaders as nurturing, caring, and intimate; it also is consistent in its contrast to descriptions of male leaders as valuing autonomy, objectivity, and fairness. Rosener's work also supports men's tendency to use the power of their position in transactional exchanges (e.g., exchanging rewards for services rendered or punishment for poor performance).

These differences are supported by Helgesen (1990a), whose research revealed several dimensions where women offer perspectives and reflect values that are a source of their uniqueness and their strength. Women, she says, value "an attention to process instead of a focus on the bottom line; a willingness to look at how an action will affect other people instead of simply asking, 'What's in it for me?'; a concern for the wider needs of the community; a disposition to draw on personal, private sphere experience when dealing in the public realm; an appreciation of diversity; [and] an outsider's impatience with rituals and symbols of status that divide people who work together and so reinforce hierarchies" (pp. xx–xxi).

In the continuation of his seminal work on megatrends, Naisbitt (1982) partnered with a female forecaster to address 10 "new directions" for the 1990s (Naisbitt & Aburdene, 1990). One of the trends they predicted for the last decade of the twentieth century was that it would be the "decade of women in leadership" (p. 216).

These authors asserted that as individuals and organizations continue to evolve, they are demanding true leadership—leadership that respects people, encourages individuals to grow and contribute significantly, inspires commitment, and "empower[s] people by sharing authority" (p. 219). The individual who will provide this kind of leadership is a "self-developer" (a term initially proposed by Maccoby, 1981), "an individual who values independence, dislikes bureaucracies, and seeks to balance work with other priorities like family and recreation" (Naisbitt & Aburdene, 1990, p. 221), as well as a "teacher, facilitator, and coach" (p. 227). Women, these authors say, are extremely well positioned to function in such roles.

> "A true leader has the confidence to stand alone, the courage to make tough decisions, and the compassion to listen to the needs of others. He does not set out to be a leader, but becomes one by the quality of his actions and the integrity of his intent. In the end, leaders are much like eagles ... they don't flock, you find them one at a time."
>
> —Anonymous

Women have made important contributions to how we think about the way organizations can and should work. For example, women-run organizations often reflect a "web" structure (Helgesen, 1990a, 1990b), rather than a pyramid or typical hierarchical one.

Helgesen (1990a) reports that the women in business whom she had studied tended to disdain the hierarchical ladder and create webs rather than pyramids. In these webs, the leader is in the center of things, rather than at the top, which these women perceived as "a lonely and disconnected position" (p. 13). Webs allow everyone in the organization to be connected by invisible strands that emanate from the central goal or mission, and they value affiliation and win/win situations instead of intense competition and win/lose situations. In such a structure, "talent is nurtured and encouraged rather than commanded, . . . a variety of interconnections exist, influence and persuasion take the place of giving orders, . . . the lines of authority are less defined, [there is more dependence] upon a moral center, [and] compassion, empathy, inspiration, and direction" (p. 225) all play significant roles. Finally, webs allow the group to take full advantage of every person's talents and skills, permit a more effective exchange of information, and minimize conflicts that arise from misunderstanding or lack of communication.

This type of "connective leadership" (Lipman-Blumen, 1992) is endorsed as a style that "fits" with today's organizations. It incorporates networking, relationship building, empowerment, and mutual responsibilities among the leader and followers.

Leadership in this kind of organization encourages interdependence, increased involvement of all members of the group, communication, and consensus, all of which are needed in the chaotic world of today and tomorrow. Helgesen (1990a,1992) asserts that women possess the skills, perspectives, and values needed to engage in this type of leadership. Indeed, in contrast to the Great Man Theory of leadership, which claims that some men are born leaders, Weddington (1991) asserts that "some leaders are born women." One would expect, therefore, that women will emerge from the twentieth century in stronger positions of leadership.

Combining the Best of "Femaleness" and "Maleness"

Schein (1989) cautions us to be careful when talking about "feminine leadership" and says that the assumption that women lead differently than men is dangerous and perpetuates sex role stereotyping. She reports that research shows more differences within each sex than between the sexes, noting that "as individuals, executive women and men seem to be virtually identical psychologically, intellectually and emotionally" (Morrison, White, & Velsor as cited in Schein, 1989, p. 156). However, this author does suggest that women might lead differently if our organizational systems were changed, and she urges America's corporate executives to restructure the work setting so that work and family are no longer separate but interface, a model similar to the one that exists in Norway and is quite successful. For example, if either parent needs to pick children up at school in the afternoon, the work day is structured to accommodate this "out of the office" responsibility.

In a work setting that values both career and family and that is more understanding of and willing to struggle with accommodating this interface, women would be likely to be more successful (Schein, 1989). In light of women's tendency to prefer "webs" to "pyramids" in the work setting and in other arenas (Helgesen, 1990a, 1990b) and the growing number of women-run businesses that reflect this organizational approach, we may, indeed, see the emergence of women as major players in making significant changes in our society, as Naisbitt and Aburdene (1990) suggested.

The new leadership paradigm that is emerging and will continue to be needed in the complex, chaotic future calls for individuals who facilitate interaction among leaders and followers, who empower followers, and who can successfully combine "maleness" and "femaleness" as an androgynous leader (Cann & Siegfried, 1990; Lipman-Blumen, 1992; Schein, 1989). The androgynous leader blends dominance, assertiveness, and competitiveness—all of which are needed in a world where resources are increasingly limited—with concern for relationships, cooperativeness, and humanitarian values, which also are needed in a world characterized by chaos, uncertainty, and ambiguity. Table 6–2 suggests what women and men both need to do to be androgynous.

Women do think and act differently than men, and nurses have a perspective that is different than that of physicians. Instead of this being something we should apologize for, however, or something women and nurses should try to change, it is something we should applaud. The differences also are something both men and women should exploit and use to benefit the patients, families, and communities to whom we provide care. By combining the best of "female leadership" and "male leadership," our visions can be more clearly articulated and better communicated, we can be more effective in guiding change, we can enhance the abilities of followers, we can strengthen our organizations, we can improve patient care, and the nursing profession can become more powerful.

The humanitarian qualities that women leaders tend to possess need to be guarded carefully against erosion; however, the pragmatic orientations that male leaders tend to possess cannot be ignored. In an age when resources are increasingly scarce and competition reigns, organizations and professions must be focused, firm, bottom line–oriented, and realistic. In such a "pragmatic age" (Fuller, 1979), however, when any means may be used to reach the desired end (e.g., reducing standards to fill positions, failing to encourage self-care in patients so that they remain dependent, and cutting professional staff to make the bottom line look healthier), it is increasingly important that humanistic leadership be exercised.

Thus, the successful leader of the future will be one who combines stereotypical "maleness" with stereotypical "femaleness," recognizing the strengths of both perspectives. To focus on one to the exclusion of the other will not benefit the individuals, organizations, or professions involved.

> *"Don't accept the dictates and little boxes that say, 'This is how the world operates.' You really have to push outside the hierarchy."*
> —Vera Martinez

Strategies for Women and Men to Be Successful Leaders in the Future

In his initial examination of the trends that seemed to be shaping our lives, Naisbitt (1982) did not address the female/male phenomenon, suggesting, perhaps, that in 1982, women were not thought to be a significant force in shaping the future of our society. In subsequent writings (Naisbitt & Aburdene, 1990), however, the role of

Table 6–2 *Becoming Androgynous*

For women to be androgynous, they need to:	For men to be androgynous, they need to:
• Be powerful and forthright and have a direct, visible impact on others.	• Give evidence of how and why their lives are men's lives.
• Be entrepreneurial.	• Understand how men value women—as validators of masculinity, as a haven from the competitive male world, as the expressive partner in the relationship.
• State their own needs and refuse to back down.	
• Recognize the equal importance of accomplishing the task, as well as being concerned about the relationship.	• Be aware of how physical and political power determine behavior.
• Build support systems with other women.	• Openly express feelings of love, fear, anger, pain, joy, loneliness, and dependency.
• Be able to intellectualize and generalize.	• Personalize experience as opposed to relying on objectivity and rationality.
• Deal directly with anger and blame, thereby rejecting feelings of suffering and victimization. Be invulnerable to destructive feedback.	• Build support systems with other men, sharing competencies without competition, sharing feelings and needs.
• Talk and cry at the same time.	• Learn how to fail at a task without feeling one has failed as a man.
• Respond directly with "I" statements rather than "you" statements.	
• Be analytical and systematic and share abstract models.	• Value an identity that is not so totally defined by work.
• Take more risks with power.	• Assert the right to work for self-fulfillment rather than to play the role of provider.
• Continue to be supportive and passionate, as well as becoming more autonomous and independent.	• Listen empathetically and actively without feeling responsible for problem solving.
	• Enjoy friendship with both men and women.

women became more prominent and even became the subject of a trends book in and of itself (Aburdene & Naisbitt, 1992).

Thus, we are increasingly aware of the significance women have in shaping the future of our world. We also are increasingly sensitive to the different perspectives women and men "bring to the table." What we also need to be fully aware of, however, are the strides being made by both genders to maintain their uniqueness while at the same time incorporating characteristics of the other.

According to Gordon (1991), "women do not change the world by becoming more like men" (p. 15) and giving up the "female perspective" totally. Instead, they must work to "create a much needed sense of collaboration and community within the work-place" (p. 285) and other settings so that feminine values can be practiced alongside masculine values.

To become influential leaders and effective agents of social change, women—and men—will need to engage in individual and collective action. The following strategies may be helpful as women and men pursue leadership goals, particularly because many women—because they do approach leadership roles differ-ently from men—lack self-confidence in that role (Farley, 1999):

- Participate fully in the mainstream of broad social and politi-cal activity, as well as in arenas of power and influence. Do not allow yourself to be isolated.
- Abandon your self-image and the public image of powerless-ness and helplessness. Do not be naive about the realities of power and its uses.
- Refuse to align yourself with the culturally stereotypical female or male expectations. Do not let your need to achieve be sublimated to your need to nurture and serve, or vice versa.
- Continue to advance your education. The nurse influentials in Vance's (1977) study listed scholarship and intelligence as the most important attributes needed by nurse leaders of the future, qualities that are still seen as critically important.
- Do not allow yourself to be affected by the "impostor syn-drome" (Harvey, 1985; The Impostor Syndrome, 1986), a phenomenon common to women (Goleman, 1985; Jacobs, 1985). Instead, both women and men must believe that they have achieved success because of their skills and talents, not because of some "fluke" or because of sheer luck.
- Develop collective strategies for action. Engage in team-work and be willing to help others rather than distrusting them and seeing them as competitors, disaffiliating from each other, devaluing alliances, and seemingly wanting to "go it alone."

- Be politically and intellectually astute.
- Get involved in decision-making and policy-making boards.
- Be goal-directed, and include "providing leadership to achieve a vision" among those goals.
- Take advantage of the positive leadership traits you possess. Acknowledge those strengths.
- Assure others of your competence by earning the right credentials and receiving competitive job offers and outside acclaim.
- Learn how to give and receive help from men or women without having those interactions become sexual encounters.
- Dress powerfully, not like someone of no importance.
- Take a visible seat at meetings and participate actively.
- Seek assignments to ensure that "the woman's (or man's) point of view" is represented.
- Seek mentor relationships or apprenticeships with others who have been successful in exercising leadership. Women may particularly want to seek other women as mentors.
- Be sure that others know of your accomplishments and achievements.
- Develop a positive sense of yourself and your abilities.
- Be supportive of others, but be careful not to take on their responsibilities.
- Develop your own support systems.
- Take a stand rather than "play it safe."
- Shape your world rather than just fit into it.
- Make your presence felt.
- Be proactive. Position yourself and get prepared to take advantage of opportunities that present themselves or that you might create.
- Act based on power and choice, not based on fear.
- Learn confrontation skills and how to manage conflict effectively.
- Know yourself—your strength, your vulnerabilities, your goals, and so on.
- Develop teamwork experiences for others (e.g., students, staff nurses).
- Take charge of your own destiny.

> *"The best way to predict the future is to create it."*
> —Yogi Berra

CONCLUSION

In her examination of "The 100 Most Influential Women of All Time," Felder (1996) noted that these women—who were more likely to be writers and social reformers than scientists—have had a great and long-lasting "historical and cultural impact, have inspired us, and . . . have much to teach us about past and present culture, society, and selfhood" (pp. ix–x). She asserts the "indisputable significance of women's past, present, and future contributions to the world" (p. x). Thus women need to take pride in the unique role they can play in providing leadership.

Women and men both need to hold onto the strength of their uniqueness but, at the same time, incorporate talents typically exhibited by the other. In other words, a movement toward more androgynous leadership and organizations that combine the benefits of hierarchies with those of "webs" may be most effective for the individuals in those groups or organizations, the individuals and communities they serve, and the professions they represent.

Critical Thinking 6–1

Critical Thinking Exercises

Observe a female nurse and a male nurse in interaction with patients, physicians, and each other. What do you notice about the similarities between their communication and interpersonal styles? What particular differences do you notice regarding what seems to be important to each, what values each conveys in his or her communications and actions, how each approaches a problem or conflict, and so on? How do your observations compare with the differences discussed here?

Think about your own childhood and current situation. What were some of the "rules" by which you were expected to behave? Were those rules made explicit to you, or were they merely implied or suggested? What differences, if any, do you recall about how boys and girls behaved in grammar school and high school and what each group seemed to value? Do you think your experiences were fairly typical? If so, what can you conclude about how parents, schools, and the larger society socialize boys and girls into stereotypical roles?

Select one of the women listed in Felder's (1996) book (e.g., Eleanor Roosevelt, Margaret Sanger, Harriet Tubman, Rosa Parks) and read a more extensive biography about her. To what extent did she reflect the characteristics of women leaders discussed in this chapter? To what extent did she also incorporate "masculine leadership" behaviors to be more androgynous? What strategies can you identify from this analysis that might help you be more effective as a leader?

Write a poem of 20 lines or less that conveys the essence of the strength of "feminine leadership" and that of "masculine leadership." Now read that poem out loud. Given all that you have read and thought about this topic and all the many things you could have said, what points were most significant to you that you absolutely had to include them in your 20 lines? Why do you think these points are so significant to you?

_____

_____

References

Aburdene, P., & Naisbitt, J. (1992). *Megatrends for women*. New York: Villard Books.

American Association of University Women. (1992). *How schools shortchange girls. Executive summary.* Washington, DC: American Association of University Women.

Brooks, A. (1983). For the woman: Strides and snags. *New York Times,* October 16, 1983, p. 31.

Cann, A., & Siegfried, W.D. (1990). Gender stereotypes and dimensions of effective leader behavior. *Sex Roles 23*(7/8), 413–419.

Farley, S. (1999). Leadership. In R.C. Swansburg & R.J. Swansburg (Eds.), *Introductory management and leadership for nurses: An interactive text* (2nd ed.). Boston: Jones & Bartlett.

Felder, D.G. (1996). *The 100 most influential women of all time: A ranking past and present.* New York: Citadel Press.

Fuller, S. (1979). Humanistic leadership in a pragmatic age. *Nursing Outlook 27*(12), 770–773.

Goleman, D. (1985). Feeling like a fake. *The Executive Female 8*(5), 34–37.

Gordon, S. (1991). *Prisoners of men's dreams. Striking out for a new feminine future.* Boston: Little, Brown.

Grunwald, L. (1992). If women ran America. *Life 15*(6), 36–46.

Harvey, J.C. (1985). *If I'm so successful, why do I feel like a fake? The impostor syndrome.* New York: Pocket Books.

Helgesen, S. (1990a). *The female advantage: Women's ways of leadership.* New York: Doubleday Currency.

Helgesen, S. (1990b). The pyramid and the web. *The New York Times Forum,* May 27, 1990, p. 13.

Helgesen, S. (1992). Feminism and nursing—"Feminine principles" of leadership: The perfect fit for nursing. *Revolution: The Journal of Nurse Empowerment 2*(2), 50–57, 135.

The impostor syndrome. (1986). *Management Solutions 31*(8), 18–19.

Jacobs, S. (1985). How businesswomen overcome a malady—"Impostor syndrome." *New England Business 7*(E), 66–67.

Kram, K.E., & Hampton, M.M. (1998). When women lead. The visibility-vulnerability spiral. In E.B. Klein, F. Gabelnick, & P. Herr (Eds.), *The psychodynamics of leadership* (pp. 193–218). Madison, CT: Psychosocial Press.

Levenstein, A. (1981). Leadership and Sex. *Supervisor Nurse 12*(1), 15–16.

Lipman-Blumen, J. (1992). Connective leadership: Female leadership styles in the 21st century workplace. *Sociological Perspectives 35*(1), 183–203.

Long, S. (1998). Discourse and corporate leadership. Transformation by or of the feminine? In E.B. Klein, F. Gabecnick, & P. Herr (Eds.), *The psychodynamics of leadership* (pp. 219–245). Madison, CT: Psychological Press.

Maccoby, M. (1981). *The leader: A new face for American management.* New York: Simon and Schuster.

Melia, J., & Lyttle, P. (1986). *Why Jenny can't lead: Understanding the male dominant system.* Saguache, CO: Communication Creativity.

Naisbitt, J. (1982). *Megatrends: Ten new directions transforming our lives.* New York: Warner Books.

Naisbitt, J., & Aburdene, P. (1990). *Megatrends 2000: Ten new directions for the 1990's.* New York: William Morrow & Co.

Rosener, J. (1990). Ways women lead. *Harvard Business Review 68*(6), 19–24.

Schein, V.E. (1989). Would women lead differently? In W.E. Rosenbach & R.L. Taylor (Eds.), *Contemporary issues in leadership* (2nd ed.) (pp. 154–160). Boulder, CO: Westview Press.

Sexes differ on military force. (1985). *Higher Education and National Affairs 34*(23), 7.

Stivers, C. (1991). Why can't a woman be less like a man? Women's leadership dilemma. *Journal of Nursing Administration 21*(5), 47–51.

Vance, C.N. (1977). *A group profile of contemporary influentials in American nursing.* Unpublished doctoral dissertation, Teachers College, Columbia University, New York.

Vance, C.N. (1979). Women leaders: Modern day heroines or social deviants? *Image 11*(2), 37–41.

Weddington, S. (1991). Some leaders are born women (The Novello Lecture). Paper presented at the National League for Nursing Convention, Nashville, TN, June 11, 1991.

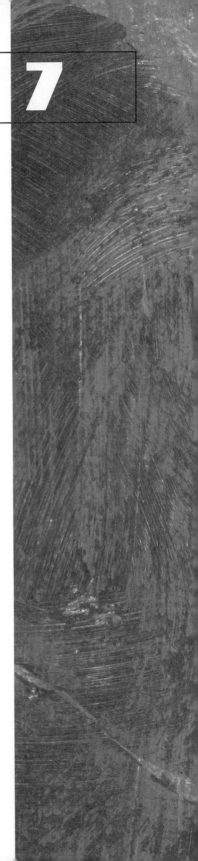

CHAPTER 7

Chaos and Disequilibrium

Invigorating, Challenging, and Growth-Producing

Chaos and Disequilibrium

Invigorating, Challenging, and Growth-Producing

Learning Objectives

☐ Describe the process by which leaders and followers can thrive and grow despite the chaos of the healthcare system.

☐ Describe how chaos can propel individuals and organizations to accomplish goals.

☐ Analyze how nurse leaders can use the change process effectively in the realization of a vision.

☐ Formulate strategies that decrease resistance to change.

☐ Describe how purposeful introduction of conflict can generate change.

INTRODUCTION

Surviving tumultuous "white water" of the current healthcare system—with its redesign, "rightsizing," and increased emphasis on cost containment—is a tremendous challenge for nurses and other healthcare providers, as well as for patients and families, communities, and organizations. Providers must create new systems, partner more effectively with each other and with patients, and work cohesively to provide cost-effective quality care and achieve desired patient outcomes. They also need to change the way they think about care and consider the patient's whole health status, not merely separate illness episodes.

As we move from the Scientific (or Newtonian) Age to the Relationship (or New Leadership) Age, nurses must incorporate a new perspective: that chaos is a good thing because it is what makes us evolve and grow. New nursing leaders need to be willing to make educated guesses, use their intuition, and be comfortable with uncertainty and ambiguity, not merely rely on formulas that a computer may generate from patient acuity codes. Nurses must take the time to develop their leadership ability so that they can be the moving force of nursing's evolution, thereby creating our preferred future. As nurses we can no longer remain as we are today. We must develop adaptive skills to manage conflict, the ability to effectively delegate to other healthcare workers, creativity to develop new caring strategies, maturity to recognize our lifelong learning needs, and the astuteness to position ourselves in arenas where significant decisions are being made. In other words, it is time to stop merely "talking the talk" and time to begin "walking the walk."

Adjusting the Leader Role and the Practice of Leadership

Nurses must acclimate themselves to feelings of uneasiness, ambiguity, and the unknown. By applying quantum theory principles (Porter-O'Grady, 1998a), we can realize that all systems work from inside out, not from top down or bottom up; relationship is as significant as control in maintaining effectiveness. Although systems cannot be predicted with certainty, we know that tension between stability and chaos creates change. The new leader, therefore, must do the following:

- Stand on the edge of previous knowledge and ability (Dreher, 1996, p. 5).
- Transform problems into solutions.
- Be a part of a universe that never stands still (p. 13).
- Realize that the ability to adapt to change is more important than being specialized in a field.
- Be able to help others resolve and grow from conflict.

"Use the constant change around you as your opportunity to change people's perceptions of you, and to prove your skills and ability to contribute."

—Susan Rehwaldt and
Mary Lou Higgerson

Leaders must focus more on cooperation than on competition (Dreher, 1996, p. 228).

Definition of Chaos

Chaos, or extreme, unpredictable disorganization and surprise, is most apparent in the world today. Wheatley and Kellner-Rogers (1996) remind us that a "system maintains itself only if change is occurring somewhere in it all the time" (p. 33). So one must view chaos or disorder as a means to survival. In other words, if there were no arguments or differences of opinion, the status quo would be maintained and there would be no individual growth. In addition, organizational survival would be threatened. The following questions were posed by Wheatley (1992, p. 73) to people who tend to believe that everything has to have a place and be labeled and filed away: "Why would we stay locked in our belief that 'truth' exists in objective form? Why would we stay locked in our belief that there is one right way to do something, or one correct interpretation to a situation, when the universe welcomes diversity and seems to thrive on a multiplicity of meanings? Why would we avoid participation and worry only about its risks? Why would we resist the rich visions and strong futures that emerge when we come together to create the world? Why would we ever choose rigidity or predictability when we have been invited to be part of the generative processes of the cosmos?"

Questions such as these invite one to discard old ways and embrace chaos theory. Many creative, motivated, and enthusiastic individuals thrive on chaos and are most successful in their personal and professional lives, despite an incredibly confusing climate. Others may become depressed and wallow in the disorder

(Wheatley, 1992). For example, some nurses who are temporarily assigned to a different unit see that situation as an opportunity to expand their knowledge, skills, and networks. However, other nurses get angry with having to work on a different unit and may become so absorbed with that anger that they cannot rise to the assignment, barely maintain safety, and complain to anyone who will listen, including patients and their families. Is it this latter group of nurses' insecurities, fear of the unknown, or inability to deal with change that prevents them from turning what is seen as a bad situation into something positive? If situations such as these were to be seen as opportunities for learning new things, fear of the unknown could be minimized as these nurses learn the clinical skills and clinical decision making associated with the new unit's patient population. As a result, they would grow more confident and increase their ability to survive the "chaos" associated with having to work on different units.

This "negative energy" also could be refocused by conducting patient rounds in which nurses share their approaches to caring for a patient. With this dialog, new and experienced nurses could learn a great deal from each other. Indeed, when everyone and everything can link together, systems form that can create more possibilities for all. "This is why life organizes, why life seeks systems . . . so that more may flourish" (Wheatley & Kellner-Rogers, 1996, p. 19).

Chaos in Nursing

In the Newtonian era, the leader was expected to help organizations adapt to change by establishing goals, obtaining commitment to the goals from employees at all levels in the bureaucracy, and decreasing uncertainty (Porter-O'Grady, 1995, p. 342). The assumptions that guided these behaviors of leaders and managers and, unfortunately, the educators of healthcare leaders included the following (Porter-O'Grady, 1995, p. 342):

- If something works once, keep trying it.
- If employees' needs are identified, managers can manipulate them to improve the organization but not necessarily the employee.
- Large effects have large causes.
- Each employee should confine himself or herself to his or her specific job description.
- Given the organizational structure, one should know that lines of authority and information flow are similar.

One can see that this view emphasized more of a management focus on planning and controlling, rather than a leadership focus on empowering the group. With the new leadership paradigm, one must realize that individuals are more effective leaders when they can keep their organization on the edge of confusion because it is only then that the whole organization can grow in a creative and productive fashion.

The uncertainty of healthcare flows from the quantum and chaotic nature of the world over time. Therefore, we should stop trying to plan every step and predict each happening. Indeed, we must realize that we can never come close to knowing all there is to know about a topic or planning every step. "The universe is no longer seen as made up of a multitude of objects, but as one invisible dynamic whole with interrelated parts which can be understood only as a pattern of a cosmic process" (McDaniel, 1998, p. 343). Hence we have to accept that no matter how much we know about the world, there are far more questions than there are answers!

Nurses also have to realize that the lengthy "to-do" task lists they routinely develop at the beginning of a workday can be nothing more than skeletal frameworks because such lists cannot possibly encompass all that nurses will need to do that day. Being extremely task-oriented and using a minute-to-minute structure to organize one's work must give way to critically thinking out new problems. Because of the exceptional complexity of the nurse role today, organizational charts, time management lists, and critical pathways have served almost as survival techniques by giving some structure in a highly chaotic environment. Unfortunately, to-do lists and predictive pathways inhibit our ability to see things globally. Nurses must stop trying to block out the chaos of the healthcare delivery system and instead embrace it.

Complexity of the Registered Nurse Role in the Current Healthcare System

What seems to be key to succeeding in this ever-changing time is having the ability to appreciate the interrelationships among multiple variables. For example, when a new managed care system takes effect, several chronically ill patients may be forced to transfer to another primary care provider. Now no patient-provider relationship exists, and all involved parties must begin all over again. In addition, it probably will take more time for the new provider to care for these complex patients, compared with the original provider, because he or she does not know the patient. Therefore, the payer will have to pay for more visits, the patient has to worry about getting to the new office and building trust with the new provider, and the patient and provider will have to invest energy into starting a new relationship.

Many healthcare agencies and institutions have experienced redesign either through downsizing, merging, or acquisition. Nurse leaders must avoid some of the pitfalls that have occurred. Seago (1997, pp. 49–50) describes some of the problems and suggests what nurses can do to avoid them:

- Nurses need to slow down with any changes and not attempt to make multiple changes at the same time.
- Nurses need to involve (i.e., be proactive and network with) the major players such as physicians and other healthcare workers, because if everyone knew the possible ramifications of decreasing professional staff in the community agency or on the clinical units, some of the drastic cuts would perhaps not be made.
- Nurse managers must be very involved in their agency's day-to-day work and remain cognizant of the challenges of each shift or day's assignments.
- All staff members must be trained appropriately and then be held accountable for doing their work.
- All measures to evaluate outcomes must be well-defined.

Facilitating Leadership in Chaos

Tonges (1997) suggests the following principles for succeeding where chaos reigns:

- Stay informed.
- Know and be guided by your values.
- Learn and use new technology.
- Accept and work with change.
- Renew yourself.

Neubauer (1998) agrees with these principles and recommends that people concentrate on renewing themselves, a process she defines as continuous self-assessment, being aware of one's own reactions, obtaining feedback, caring for oneself, and setting goals. Leaders also should use diverse work teams to brainstorm solutions and create vision, focus on ongoing learning and the continued development of critical thinking skills, and use effective communication skills. Further suggestions for providing strategic leadership in uncertain times are enumerated by McDaniel (1998, pp. 358–361):

- Stop planning and being preoccupied with order so that you can learn to cope with the unknowable.
- Move to the edge of chaos in order to find creative and new directions.
- Expect many people to be leaders because this will make for a vibrant organization.

- Allow for autonomy and small fluctuations so that people can learn to adapt and adjust to change.
- Improve the connections between colleagues because "the quality of connections between workers is more important than the quality of each individual" (p. 359).
- Do not allow people to say "That's not my job"—teach them what other people are doing.
- Assist peers to become "skilled at handling ambiguous issues, revealing differences, and generating new perspectives" (p. 360).
- Assist organizations and people to discover goals themselves.
- Work smarter, not necessarily harder.
- Provide for the emergence of vision.

> *"Vision is the art of seeing things invisible."*
> —Jonathan Swift

It is wise to realize that no matter how much energy is spent trying to lead through chaos, the stability one might long for is not really the solution at all because stability will only dampen the potential growth that may evolve if some chaos remains.

Change

It has been said that the only permanent thing in society is change. As humans, one of the most pervasive and significant concepts affecting our lives is that of change—change that comes about through our own development and maturation, change that takes place as a result of our education and our interactions with others, change that is imposed on us from outside sources, and change that we impose on ourselves and others. If we are to cope effectively with change and use it to our advantage, we must be able to recognize when it occurs, when it needs to occur, how to facilitate it, how it can be blocked, and the impact various changes and change strategies have on individuals and groups.

> *"Nothing endures but change."*
> —Heraclitus

Change is the making of something that is different from the way it was. It is an alteration; it results from differences and conflicts in a system, from information, or sometimes from unfulfilled needs. Change potentiates or allows the possibility of accomplishment of goals. It can be planned or it may be an unexpected result of a decision or other event. Change can evolve over time, or it can be a spontaneous, revolutionary occurrence. Change in one's personal and professional life can involve a transition period, during which adjustment may be successful or not. No matter what the change, a true change does not affect only a single person; instead, it permeates the ambiance of a setting or a being and triggers some type of change in anyone who comes in contact with the individual or setting that changed.

Belasco (1990) says organizations are similar to elephants in that they both learn through conditioning. He describes this phenomenon with the following illustration (p. 2):

Trainers shackle young elephants with heavy chains to deeply embedded stakes. In that way the elephant learns to stay in its place. Older elephants never try to leave even though they have the strength to pull the stake and move beyond. Their conditioning limits their movements with only a small metal bracelet around their foot—attached to nothing.

Like powerful elephants, many companies are bound by conditioned constraints. "We've always done it this way" is as limiting to an organization's progress as the unattached chain around the elephant's foot.

It is time we move the nursing profession forward by listening to new ideas and trying new ways of doing things. We have to start "dancing" rather than feel chained to an invisible stake in the ground, and we need to start paving our own roads to our dreams. Many people often remark that they would change their lives dramatically if they could, and they say the change would focus more on self-respect and increasing quality family and friend time versus gaining power and affluence.

It seems that many people are dissatisfied with their lives but do not know how to change. They have, in a sense, been conditioned to accept their lot in life and truly are ignorant about drifting away from their routine—no matter how uncomfortable or dissatisfying it has become. Perhaps by better understanding some principles of change (Box 7–1) we can be more willing to engage in it and change our lives.

The Leader as a Change Agent

As nurses acquire new abilities and transform themselves to be leaders, they need to demonstrate great courage by sharing decision-making "power" and not feeling they have to have the last word about issues. Decisions about quality of clinical outcomes, work content, and performance effectiveness of workers will be more readily incorporated if they belong to the nurses and not just to the manager. Likewise, the staff members, having been empowered by the leader, are the ones responsible for their own practice—not the nurse manager. The days of "my nurses are such good workers" and "I need one more RN for the Saturday

> *"The secret to leadership is ... to think of your position as an opportunity to serve, not as a trumpet call to self-importance."*
>
> —J. Donald Walters

Box 7–1 *Principles of Change*

- A change in one part affects other parts and other systems.
- People affected by the change should participate in making the change.
- People should be informed of the reasons for the change.
- Concrete and specific feedback about the process of change will enhance its acceptance.
- People need assistance in dealing with the effects of the change.
- People's suggestions and contributions about the implementation of change should be sought and incorporated.
- A change must be reinforced or the system will revert to its old practices.
- Conflict may occur at any step during the change process.
- The more compatible the new ideas are with one's values and needs, the more easily a change will be adopted.
- The more trust one has in the initiator of change, the more likely one is to support the change.
- One's past experience with change can profoundly affect one's willingness to support a new idea.

eleven-to-seven shift, can't you do me a favor and work a double?" must come to an end. It is not the nurse manager's unit but the staff's. In fact, the "power" of the nurse manager will not be diminished—and may actually increase—when he or she empowers others to make change.

Kouzes and Posner (1995) believe that leaders do not always seek the challenges and consequential ramifications of change that occur but that these challenges seek the leaders. They also believe that challenge is the motivating milieu for excellence. They have found through their research that "ordinary" men and women are able to accomplish extraordinary feats, and those who function as leaders in the group realize they have skills they never knew they had, such as dealing with change (p. 53).

Two very important skills for a leader to exercise when involved in change are coaching and team building. *Coaching* is the ability to facilitate others' understanding of themselves and their abilities. It is the process by which one person (the coach—the leader) helps others understand that answers to questions or solutions to problems lie within themselves. *Team building* is the process of forming a group whose members work collegially for a common goal. Team building enhances the identification of more diversified opinions and alternatives; it fosters a more cooperative relationship among all members of the team, and it is essential to increase participation in decision making.

The new leadership is about forming relationships and connecting with others to challenge the old, bureaucratic organizational structure and old ways of doing things. Ashmos (1998) describes some conventional assumptions about the use of teams and offers suggestions of new perspectives on those old ideas (Table 7–1).

The delay in committing to a decision allows team members to discuss the issue fully and explore all possible options. Unlearning requires giving up old behaviors so that new ones may be taken on, and it undoubtedly will cause conflict; however, when this conflict is addressed, feelings surface and the ultimate outcome will be better. It is obvious that as team members discuss and argue various points of view, turmoil in the organization will occur. Rather than being distressed by this turmoil, however, leaders are excited by it because it is exactly what the organization needs if it is to be successful. Teams are going to constantly cause change(s) in the organization's strategy by incorporating the outcomes of their discussions. Undermining the existing hierarchy and challenging the organization's belief system are necessary components to prevent an organization from maintaining the status quo. When an individual, group, community, or team is able to empower itself, effective leadership has occurred, positive change is likely, and the organization can grow tremendously. With this new perspective, the importance of developing self-directed teams in any organization is made abundantly clear.

Facilitating the Change Process

Leaders are necessary to facilitate change. The environment must be ripe or made ripe, there must be a reason for the change to occur, the players must be willing to try to change, and the change must yield growth—positive or negative. Nurses must be willing to try to think in a new way despite the multiple barriers to change that we confront.

Table 7-1 *The Use of Teams*	
Conventional Assumptions	**New Perspectives**
Teams encourage commitment and acceptance of decisions.	Effective teams delay commitment and acceptance of decisions.
Teams help the organization by gathering necessary information for making decisions.	Effective teams help the organization "unlearn" and then relearn.
Teams help create order in organizations.	Effective teams help create disorder in organizations.
Teams enable execution of the organization's strategy.	Effective teams alter the organization's strategy.
Teams support and reinforce the hierarchy.	Effective teams undermine the hierarchy.
Teams are guided by the organization's belief.	Effective teams challenge the organization's belief.
Teams are empowered by top management.	Effective teams empower themselves.

Source: Ashmos, D. (1998). Building effective healthcare teams. In W.J. Duncan, P.M. Ginter, & L.E. Swayne (Eds.), *Handbook of healthcare management* (pp. 313–337). Malden, MA: Blackwell.

Knox and Irving (1997) studied nurse managers' ($N = 15$) perceptions of healthcare executives' behavior during organizational change and rank-ordered those perceptions (Table 7–2). The findings of this study reinforce the importance of effective communication, recognition of staff welfare as well as patient safety during a transition, and empowerment of staff to accomplish the processes necessary for the change to evolve. These rankings can assist nurses in any position to facilitate the change process.

There is no doubt that effective change requires leadership. However, both leaders and followers must be motivated and energized to implement positive changes and thrive in the chaotic healthcare world of today. Perhaps all nurses must assess their ability to respond to change. The Readiness-to-Change Quotient (Fig. 7–1) is one way to stimulate nurses' thinking about how they can shape future changes in healthcare and how open their

(Text continued on page 149.)

Table 7–2	Results of Nurse Managers' Rankings of Healthcare Executives' Behavior during Change
Ranking	**Behavior**
1	Frequent communication of plans and progress during the transition
2	High visibility on work units during the organizational change
3	Verbalized commitment within the institution for the quality of patient care during the transition
4	Verbalized commitment within the institution for staff welfare during the transition
5	Presentation of rewards and recognition for staff performance during the transition
6	Empowerment of staff to accomplish changes for which they are responsible
7	Presentation of opportunities for staff to clarify issues in a nonthreatening environment
8	Follow-up on staff suggestions and questions related to the transition
9	Offers of support and assistance for problem solving during the transition
10	Presentation of informational and educational programs before implementation

Adapted from Knox, S., & Irving, J. (1997). Nurse managers' perceptions of health-care executive behaviors during organizational change. *Journal of Nursing Administration 27*(11), 37.

Fig. 7–1 *Readiness-to-Change Quotient*

PART I: HOW READY AM I?
1 = Don't Know; 2 = Strongly Disagree; 3 = Disagree; 4 = Agree; 5 = Strongly Agree

1. I know the current status of national and state healthcare reform legislation. _____
2. I'm aware of how trends changing the healthcare system will affect my practice. _____
3. My colleagues and I on my work unit have discussed healthcare reform and its implications for our practice and our roles. _____
4. I can influence the course of change in my workplace. _____
5. Some of the changes occurring in healthcare reform are consistent with Nursing's interests and concerns. _____
6. I integrate into my practice a concern for continuity of care. _____
7. I'm greatly concerned about patients' satisfaction with the care my colleagues and I provide _____
8. Patient education is a major focus on my practice. _____
9. I've played a significant role in developing a plan for improving patient care during the past six months. _____
10. I have a plan for my own professional development to enhance my role in a changing healthcare system. _____
11. I know what my state nurses association is doing to influence health care reform. _____
12. I've communicated with one of my legislators about nursing practice issues affected by government policy. _____
13. I'm involved in community organizations, such as the school board, citizen action groups, or political parties that have an interest in healthcare reform. _____
14. I can use JCAHO standards (or those of another accrediting body) to argue for changes in my healthcare organization that will foster better patient care. _____
15. I can discuss the market forces affecting my healthcare organization and my practice. _____

TOTAL (add the above points) _____

PART II: HOW READY IS MY ORGANIZATION? (NOTE: If you work for a public health agency, school, or industry, you may need to translate some of the questions here to better fit your practice setting.)
1 = Don't Know; 2 = Strongly Disagree; 3 = Disagree; 4 = Agree; 5 = Strongly Agree

1. My organization provides programs or forums for discussion of changes and trends in healthcare delivery. _____
2. Nursing administration has developed a strategic plan for transforming nursing practice in my organization. _____
3. The staff in my organization is encouraged to be creative and to introduce innovations for improving patient care. _____
4. Patient satisfaction data are regularly shared with the staff. _____
5. Continuous quality improvement or total quality management approaches have been used to improve patient care within my organization. _____
6. Nursing is involved in decision-making about staff mix. _____
7. My organization has developed a plan for expanding ambulatory care or enhancing continuity of care. _____

(Continued)

Fig. 7–1 *Readiness-to-Change Quotient Continued*

8. My organization belongs to a larger network of healthcare delivery systems (for example, hospitals, outpatient clinics, home care agencies). _____

9. My organization is in good financial health. _____

10. My organization uses or plans to use advanced practice nurses. _____

11. My organization supports the staff's continuing education, reeducation, and advancement to help bring about changes needed in patient care. _____

12. Nurses are included on all committees in my organization involved in policy development and strategic planning. _____

13. The chief nurse officer in my organization has the authority. _____

14. My organization supports collaborative, multidisciplinary team approaches to patient care. _____

15. My organization is visibly marketing its centers of excellence to the community it serves. _____

TOTAL (add the above points) _____

DIRECTIONS: Add the number values of your answers to the statements in "How Ready am I?" (Part I), and mark on the horizontal axis of the scoring grid the point that corresponds to the total. Similarly, add the number values of your answers to the statements in "How ready is my organization?" (Part II), and mark on the vertical axis of the grid the point corresponding to that total. Then find on the grid the point whose coordinates are your two scores.

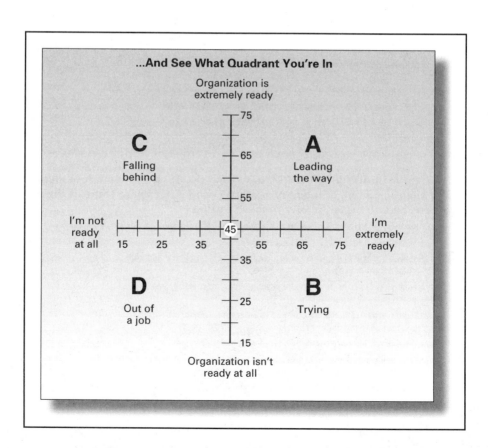

Fig. 7–1 *Readiness-to-Change Quotient Concluded*

Here's what your scores mean:

If your score places you in **Quadrant A**, congratulations. You're "leading the way" and staying abreast of changes and trends in healthcare. And you work for an organization that's well positioned to thrive in a changing environment.

If you're in **Quadrant B**, you're "trying," but either you don't know what's going on in your organization or your organization isn't doing much to inspire your confidence in its future. Ignorance is dangerous for both you and your organization. If you answered "I don't know" to many of the organization readiness questions, start to ask questions, read internal communications, and join committees that are planning the organization's future directions. If you didn't answer "I don't know" to most of those questions, your organization is in trouble—or will be soon. Given today's competitive environment, you'll need to take a hard look at whether you want to stay with your organization and have a strong enough commitment to help it move forward. You may want to assess how well other healthcare organizations in your area are poised for change and what opportunities they may offer.

If you scored in **Quadrant C**, your organization may be reconsidering its commitment to you . . . you're "falling behind." Besides getting up to date with changes in your organization, you need to look beyond your workplace, at the big picture—what's happening in healthcare today and what will be happening tomorrow.

Finally, if you scored in **Quadrant D**, you need to spend a great deal of time and energy learning about the changes in healthcare and looking for a healthier organization in your area. Chances are, you'll be "out of a job" unless your job happens to be at the only hospital or organization of its kind in the area, and it's still experiencing a shortage of nurses.

Source: Mason, D. & Leavitt, J. (1998). The revolution in healthcare: What's your readiness quotient? In E.C. Hein (Ed.). *Contemporary leadership behavior: Selected readings* (5th ed.) (pp. 452–454). Philadelphia: Lippincott.

organization is to change (Mason & Leavitt, 1998). The tool measures the individual's and the organization's readiness to change. The tool has not been tested for reliability or validity but is a parameter that can help each of us gain insight about how ready we and our organizations are for the changes confronted by healthcare today. Awareness of such "readiness-to-change quotients" will help any leader wanting to implement a change to prepare people for the change and its consequences.

The Process of Change

The current and predicted rate of change in society in general and in healthcare in particular is phenomenal. Such change requires institutions to modify their goals, organizational structure and culture, technologies, and strategic planning. Leaders are therefore faced with an inordinate amount of work, which, although very energy-consuming, also is revitalizing and rewarding for most. Leaders must help others see the need for change, work with others to implement change, evaluate the effect of change, and participate in each stage of the change process. They also must understand what people experience as they go through change.

Perhaps one of the most useful theories to help us understand this phenomenon is that espoused by Lewin in 1951. He identified three phases of change:

1. *Unfreezing,* in which people are preparing for change
2. *Moving,* in which people have accepted the need for a change and actually engage in the change
3. *Refreezing,* in which the new change is integrated into the system and becomes part of the new norm or culture

For example, a unit practicing primary nursing is experiencing turmoil related to staffing and reporting as a result of the increased acuity of patients and decreased number of registered nurses (RNs). It becomes obvious that old methods of assignment are no longer working and some unfreezing must occur. The staff and nurse manager engage in some brainstorming activities and decide, after exploring many options, to institute a charge position for each shift. Once the new charge position is started, the unit enters Lewin's moving stage and works to refine the position and its duties to make it most effective. As the unit adjusts to and incorporates the new position, refreezing, or the integration of the position into daily work, occurs. This approach to change is congruent with the new leadership style because it is a dynamic process that is planned or facilitated by the leader and followers but then also is allowed to evolve spontaneously and mesh into the system.

Whatever change theory one applies, it is important to realize that the stages of change are merely categories to help our thinking, not discrete steps that begin and end abruptly. In other words, change typically is not a clear-cut process that can be achieved by following a formula; transformational change, as noted earlier, is an evolving process that tends to be the product of a group's vision over time, and revolutionary change follows no clear-cut formula. Perhaps nursing is in the process of a revolution. It appears we have moved through the unfreezing stage and are in the process of moving toward a more autonomous role in the healthcare arena. Advanced practice nursing is taking hold in every setting of healthcare delivery, and patient outcomes are beginning to validate the significance of our contributions. RNs and hiring institutions are realizing the need for a baccalaureate degree in nursing as the staff nurse position becomes more and more integrated into the healthcare team structure. RNs and physicians are collaborating more than ever before, and patient outcomes are being tracked to identify both the nursing and medical interventions responsible for a positive or negative outcome. As outcomes become publicized, our profession must move toward the refreezing stage.

Perhaps the following "rules" for achieving change in an organization (Porter-O'Grady, 1998b) will be helpful to nurse leaders:

- *Make no exceptions.* Everyone must engage in the change process. "Organizations can no longer afford to carry those who do not or cannot support the necessary redesign" (p. 227).
- *Read the signs.* Be aware of all kinds of trends that are occurring, not just those related to healthcare. The leader must be prepared to design the future, not merely react to it.
- *Construct a vision.* "Help people find meaning in the purposes for work, not just in the work itself" (p. 229). In other words, "if organizations are to get the partnership, equity, accountability and ownership that is required for sustaining the organization, a vision must lead the way" (p. 230).
- *Empower the center.* Get those people closest to the point of service (e.g., the nurses and those who will be most affected by the change) involved in any change.
- *Construct new architecture.* "New roles and work behavior cannot be reinforced unless the organizational structure in place supports and sustains them" (p. 231).
- *Always have a plan of action.* This allows everyone to "act in concert and move in the same direction collaboratively and consistently" (p. 232).
- *Evaluate, adjust, and evaluate again.* The leader must "see the whole and not get caught up simply enumerating its parts" (p. 233).

Barriers to Change

> "There is a certain relief in change, even though it is from bad to worse; as I have found in traveling in a stage-coach, that it is often a comfort to shift one's position and be bruised in a new place."
>
> —Washington Irving

The captain of a ship steers that vessel from one port to another using carefully plotted coordinates. Why then does the ship veer off its course, sometimes miles off track of the destination? Why does the ship end up beached on a shoal not marked on the charts? Why does an iceberg cut up the ship? The answer to all these questions is that life is unpredictable, and captains must consider many other factors besides coordinates when navigating their ships. So, too, nurse leaders must consider multiple factors and anticipate potential problems when instituting changes.

Many factors can serve as barriers to change, including decreased resources, lack of support, resistance, poor communication mechanisms, or pressures to get the day-to-day work done. The more barriers there are to the change, the more effort will be needed to deal with those barriers, and consequently, the less energy will be available to institute the actual change.

Dealing with Conflict Generated by Change

Leaders work toward positive outcomes of change, but they also need to realize that there may be negative outcomes as well. However, those negative outcomes may actually be positive ones. One of the most common outcomes of change is *conflict,* something that historically has been viewed as negative but something that actually is positive. The positive results of conflict are growth, an ability to accept that what was can no longer be, and collaboration, which builds healthy relationships.

In the new science of leadership, conflict is embraced wholeheartedly because it is an instigator of change and ultimately growth. Yet, to deal with the conflict generated, some goals may be lost, the vision may be altered, and an extraordinary amount of energy may be needed as the group moves through the change. The evolution of individuals, groups, and organizations experiencing the change, however, far surpasses the time and effort involved. Dreher (1996) reminds us that the Tao says we can develop better harmony by looking for it within us—by decreasing our anxiety and defensiveness in conflict. Using the yin (patience, process, and empathy) with the yang (courage and positive action) the Tao leader balances opposites within herself or himself to augment the power of Tao.

Leaders must be confident, focused, and able to balance personal and professional goals and conflicts to succeed with orchestrating a change because only a self-actualized leader will be able to spend the energy needed to take on the challenge of change. People must have a "clear perspective and life balance" in order to lead in the face of change (Hawkins, 1998). Ultimately, it is better to choose to change and design one's own approach to change than to have a change imposed by some external force.

> *"Tentative efforts lead to tentative outcomes. Therefore give yourself fully to your endeavors. Decide to construct your character through excellent actions and determine to pay the price of a worthy goal. The trials you encounter will introduce you to your strengths. Remain steadfast ... and one day you will build something that endures, something worthy of your potential."*
>
> —Epictetus
> (Roman Teacher/Philosopher)

It is necessary for the nurse leader in organizations experiencing change to be aware of the following vulnerable stressful areas: (1) communication systems, (2) project target dates, (3) people stability, (4) cash flow, (5) effective leadership propelling the group to fulfill the organization's vision, and (6) proactive internal and external networking (Hawkins, 1998). As the change proceeds through all layers of the organization, people often experience stress in the following areas: (1) maintaining a proactive view of the future, (2) accessing mentors, (3) having a positive attitude toward the organization's atmosphere, (4) maintaining good relationships with supervisors, and (5) having pride in the organization (Hawkins, 1998).

An example that portrays these stressors is the nurse who has an extremely challenging patient assignment and is assigned an unlicensed assistive personnel (UAP), who is brand new to the job. The nurse has to spell out every detail to the UAP and cannot delegate many tasks until he or she is comfortable with the aide's work. In addition to this extra work, the RN has to orient a float RN who has his or her own separate patient assignment and has been told by the supervisor to ask the staff RN for assistance with anything about which he or she feels uncomfortable. The staff RN is likely to expend only so much energy and accept this type of working condition only so many times before experiencing stress in all five of the areas noted by Hawkins (1998). Whether the nurse stays in this job or not will depend greatly on how effectively the leader can help the nurse want to be part of the organization's future, help the nurse gain access to a mentor, get the nurse involved in the unit, provide encouragement, and help him or her maintain effective relationships with her supervisors. Leaders for the new millennium must know how to deal with change and the conflict typically associated with it.

Conclusion

There is no doubt that nurses are experiencing enormous change in their own practice and in the environments in which they practice. Leaders cannot have total control or meticulously follow short- or long-term plans in these uncertain times. This is a good thing because the chaos that exists can be used to promote extraordinary growth for the profession, the organization, and all individuals involved in it.

Leaders must have the ability to identify when they should deviate from a plan, and they must surround themselves with a diverse team. Networking, partnering, and collaborating are mandatory for nurses to practice most successfully. Coaching nurses in identifying their strengths and building self-esteem will assist in decreasing fear of the changes the profession now faces and will continue to face in the future.

Some of the most important changes leaders should strive to make are changes in educational programs toward ones that focus on learning more than on knowing, changes in incentives for bedside nurses that recognize their significant contributions and allow them to continue to develop their expertise in that role, and changes that create more opportunities for nurses to engage in collaborative efforts with their nurse colleagues and other health-care workers. As we enter the twenty-first century, it is even more important for nurses to lead and participate in change projects that reshape healthcare practices and policy. Organizations that survive in the new millennium will be ones that encourage all members of the organization to think beyond what is currently possible and continuously participate in change.

Critical Thinking 7–1

Critical Thinking Exercises

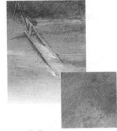

Several authors assert that resistance to change grows out of fear. Talk to your nurse colleagues about why they have resisted change. Is the bottom-line reason that of fear? If so, what seems to be feared? If not, what is the bottom-line reason given?

_____

_____

What strategies have you used or experienced being used that have resulted in reduced resistance to and a successful outcome of change?

_____

_____

Given the "state of the art" of nursing, do we need a revolution? Do your nurse colleagues agree with your position?

_____

_____

Listen to the song "The Times They Are a-Changin'" by Bob Dylan (1967). How is it that new expectations seem to emerge slowly yet still demand change?

_____

_____

Listen to the song "Revolution" by the Beatles (Lennon & McCarthy, 1968). Why would some people prefer a quicker, revolutionary approach to change?

_____

_____

Read an article about chaos in nursing in the journal *Complexity and Chaos in Nursing*. Describe how the new science of leadership correlates with how the nurse practices leadership in a state of chaos.

_____

_____

View the movie *Witness* with Harrison Ford and Alexander Goodenauf. This movie portrays how a group of people work effectively together in constructing a building. What strategies can you take from this film to apply in your job to improve group work?

_____

_____

Use a personality inventory such as the Myers-Brigg to identify your individual personality style. Discuss how the results affect your ability to communicate and to resolve and grow from conflict.

_____

_____

References

Ashmos, D. (1998). Building effective healthcare teams. In W.J. Duncan, P.M. Ginter, & L.E. Swayne (Eds.), *Handbook of healthcare management* (pp. 313–337). Malden, MA: Blackwell.

Belasco, J. (1990). *Teaching the elephant to dance: Empowering change in your organization.* New York: Crown.

Dreher, D. (1996). *The Tao of personal leadership.* New York: Harper Business.

Dylan, B. (1967). The times they are a-changin'. *Bob's Dylan's Greatest Hits,* CBS Records Inc.

Hawkins, J. (1998). *Leadership in the face of change.* www.lead-edge.com/june98.htm.

Knox, S., & Irving, J. (1997). Nurse managers' perceptions of healthcare executive behaviors during organizational change. *Journal of Nursing Administration 27*(11), 33–39.

Kouzes, J., & Posner, B. (1995). *The leadership challenge: How to keep getting extraordinary things done in organizations* (2nd ed.). San Francisco: Jossey-Bass.

Lennon, J., & McCartney, P. (1968). Revolution. *The Beatles, Past Masters,* EMI Records Ltd.

Lewin, K. (1951). *Field theory in social science: Selected theoretical papers.* New York: Harper & Row.

Mason, D. & Leavitt, J. (1998).The revolution in healthcare: What's your readiness quotient? In E.C. Hein (Ed.), *Contemporary leadership behavior: Selected readings* (5th ed.) (pp. 451–457). Philadelphia: Lippincott.

McDaniel, R. (1998). Strategic leadership: A view from quantum and chaos theories. In W.J. Duncan, P. Ginter, & L. Swayne (Eds.), *Handbook of healthcare management* (pp. 339–367). Malden, MA: Blackwell.

Neubauer, J. (1998). Thriving in chaos: Personal and career development. In E.C. Hein (Ed.), *Contemporary leadership behavior: Selected readings* (5th ed.) (pp. 247–258). Philadelphia: Lippincott.

Porter-O'Grady, T. (1998a). Quantum mechanics and the future of healthcare leadership. In E.C. Hein (Ed.), *Contemporary leadership behavior: Selected readings* (5th ed.) (pp. 403–410). Philadelphia: Lippincott.

Porter-O'Grady, T. (1998b). The seven basic rules for successful redesign. In E.C. Hein (Ed.), *Contemporary leadership behavior: Selected readings* (5th ed.) (pp. 226–235). Philadelphia: Lippincott.

Seago, J. (1997). Five pitfalls of work redesign in acute care. *Nursing Management 28*(10), 49–50.

Tonges, M. (1997). The white water of change. *Nursing Management 28*(10), 64–69, 70, 72.

Wheatley, M. (1992). *Leadership and the new science.* San Francisco: Berrett-Koehler.

Wheatley, M., & Kellner-Rogers, M. (1996). *A simpler way.* San Francisco: Berrett-Koehler.

CHAPTER 8

Shaping a Preferred Future for Nursing

Shaping a Preferred Future for Nursing

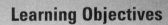

Learning Objectives

- [ ] Analyze how current societal healthcare trends can affect nursing's future.

- [ ] Examine projections for the future that are likely to have an impact on the nursing profession and healthcare.

- [ ] Describe characteristics of leaders needed to shape a preferred future for nursing.

- [ ] Propose partnerships and collaborative relationships that can help nurse leaders shape a preferred future.

- [ ] Formulate strategies that can prevent or minimize the potentially negative social, political, economic, and organizational forces that can affect the future of nursing.

- [ ] Suggest strategies whereby nurses can create our own preferred future.

INTRODUCTION

Leaders in nursing have the responsibility to prepare today for tomorrow's challenges. Although we must be fully aware of our past so that we can learn from it and we must be fully aware of our present circumstance so that we can survive in it, it is perhaps more critical that we have some sense of the future so that we can try to plan for it and shape it to our benefit. Leaders are responsible—through their vision, creativity, ability to facilitate change, and ability to manage and survive chaos—for articulating a preferred future for our profession and its practitioners, whether they be in clinical, administrative, educational, research, health policy, or other roles. Leaders, then, are responsible to help create that preferred future.

An orientation toward the future involves knowing current trends in our society and in the world; being cognizant of the social, political, economic, and organizational forces that create, influence, or are influenced by those trends; and speculating on the mutual interaction of these trends and forces with leadership needs (Naisbitt & Aburdeen, 1990; Toffler, 1990). However, leaders cannot shape the future alone; they must engage others to achieve this goal. Nursing leaders and followers must analyze scientific, technological, and healthcare trends and identify strategies to maximize the nurse's role in healthcare delivery.

Predicting the Future

When people talk about some of the things they expect to see in the twenty-first century, it often is difficult not to laugh or roll one's eyes. However, ideas that sounded like science fiction only a few years ago—gene cloning, antiaging drugs, computers, and robotics—are very real in today's world. Ideas considered "way out," unreal, or unbelievable when they were first proposed are now common. The world is changing dramatically, the "good-old days" are gone forever, and the future is happening now.

"There is only one direction for a leader: FORWARD."
—Advertisement

Kouzes and Posner (1995) recommend that we think of the future as a time for great things and that, in most instances, things will be improved. These authors surveyed leaders about the future and found that terms such as "foresight," "focus," "forecasts," "future scenarios," "perspectives," and "points of view" are common in discussions of visions of the future. It is important, however, that leaders be able to translate this language into as much detail as possible when sharing their visions so that followers can better understand what the vision represents and more fully participate in making it become a reality.

Obviously, there is no crystal ball, but there are methods that futurists can and do use to try to determine future happenings (Minkin, 1995). Leaders must know a particular area well, understand how certain occurrences in this area began and have evolved, and be knowledgeable about how patterns of related happenings might affect the area currently and in the future. This kind of information will assist the leader in knowing how and where to study trends and identify indicators of future patterns. Minkin (1995) reminds us to use past occurrences as we attempt to predict future occurrences.

Minkin (1995) also recommends using a practical approach in thinking about forecasting the future. He calls this approach TIP, which stands for trends (T), implications (I), and specific predictions (P). He describes it as examining past and current trends, contemplating the implications of these trends for one's area of interest, analyzing how the implications have changed things, and then making specific predictions as to what may occur next.

Another futurist (Moliter, 1998) recommends that leaders read the futuristic literature, review chronologies of significant developments, observe and participate in debates and forums, keep an eye open to events occurring throughout the world, and review information from the Census Bureau and the Bureau of Labor Statistics, as well as from other data sources. Every individual and every profession or group needs some context within which successful plans for the future can be made, and resources such as these help a leader create that context.

Four kinds of futures are addressed in the literature (Valiga, 1994):

1. The *probable future* is what is likely to occur if things continue as they are and no changes are made.
2. The *possible future* is what can occur if some changes are made in the current state of affairs.
3. The *plausible future* is what is likely to occur when specific efforts are made to accomplish goals.
4. The *preferred future* is what we would like to see happen.

Using this framework is a good way to brainstorm about the future. Small groups of nurses can hypothesize with scenarios, which can increase our ability to visualize what different futures might be like and strategize about how we can create the future we want for nursing. This might occur at a vision retreat where nurses engage in future forecasting and vision planning (Nanus, 1992).

Bezold (1996) offers an example of how the work of predicting future trends using scenarios can affect healthcare and the nursing profession. By analyzing changes in societal values, public policies, and individuals' behaviors that are significant to the future of health, rather than dwelling merely on medical breakthroughs, nurses can significantly influence the general welfare of humanity. For example, if society does not deal with poverty and illiteracy, both of which are related to illness, more people will use hospital emergency departments for their basic healthcare, there will be less of an emphasis on health promotion and disease prevention, and the poor are likely to have more complications of illness. If nurses become involved in developing health policy that mandates health promotion for the uninsured, impoverished, and illiterate, the people of the world are likely to have a greatly improved future.

"Leadership is a process rather than an event."

"We don't always know how, when, or what we will lead."

"Each of us wants our life to stand for something. Being able to have an impact—to make a difference—is perhaps the biggest benefit of being a leader."

—Sarah Weddington
(*Roe v. Wade* Attorney)

There are multiple areas in which nurses can make strong contributions in improving healthcare. By educating the public, providing testimony for changes in healthcare policy, and providing wellness care to the poor and underserved, nurses could significantly change the quality of life for many, as well as enhance cost savings and higher-quality health. Bezold (1996, p. 39) presents four possible scenarios of how healthcare could evolve in the future (Table 8–1).

Most nurses would probably agree that "Scenario 4: Healthy Healing Communities = Preferred Future" listed in Table 8–1 is the preferred future because it depicts a healthier, more educated population. Nurses, as leaders of health, must propel their visions forward and begin thinking in a future-forward frame to have more input into how the future will transpire.

Molitor (1998) reminds us to be aware of possible "wild cards" such as meteor strikes on earth, volcanic eruptions, or some other inconceivable event that could "throw quite a monkey wrench" into our best laid plans. We also need to realize that things no one had dreamed or thought to be so significant, such

Table 8–1 *Scenarios of Healthcare in the Future*

Scenario 1: Business as Usual = Probable Future	Healthcare increases its share of the gross national product (GNP) to 17% by 2005. Healthcare providers shift to health promotion. Poverty and lack of access to healthcare persists. The states replace the federal government in making health-care policy.
Scenario 2: Hard Times = Possible Future	A frugal system, similar to Canada's, has been adopted because of political revolt. This decreases healthcare's percentage of the GNP to 11% by 2001. Thirty percent of Americans increase their coverage to a more expensive, higher technological care so there are two healthcare systems. Therefore a "have and a have-not" system emerges.
Scenario 3: Buyer's Market = Plausible Future	High-quality healthcare services for consumers at lower costs are available. The social policies blunt inequities and lack of access for some.
Scenario 4: Healthy Healing Communities = Preferred Future	The years leading to 2010 are a time of vision and design for healthcare. All join together to pursue visions leading to improved healthcare such as annual physical exams for all children and all people over the age of 50 years, every-other-year physicals for those people between 18 and 50 years, easier access to care for chronically ill people, community and school-based health promotion centers available to all, and thorough health education for all through schools, shopping plazas, and other community centers.

Source: Adapted from Bezold, C. (1996). Your health in 2010: Four scenarios. *The Futurist 30*(5), 35–36.

as the year 2000 computer "problem," can have a significant influence on future developments.

However, this uncertainty and unpredictability is exactly what we in nursing need—something to make us think! Today's new science of leadership makes us more open to the unknown becoming a reality and accept that the future holds endless possibilities for us. It is still important, however, to attempt to shape the future or at least try to have some say in it because "foresight enhances abilities to capitalize upon opportunities, decrease adversities, gain lead time for responding and asserting leadership in trying to manage change" (Molitor, 1998, p. 59).

The future does not just happen. We dream about it and shape it to some extent every day. Whenever a change is proposed, even if it is so small it will affect only one unit or one part of an agency, that change influences the future and can contribute to the growth of the organization or profession because change of any type ultimately will have ramifications for any number of people.

"There are three kinds of people: those who make things happen; those who watch things happen; and those who wonder what happened."

—Anonymous

An example from clinical practice may help illustrate this notion of interdependence and how a change can have a "ripple effect." A nurse in the cardiothoracic intensive care unit draws on research data and suggests that every nurse use the forced warm air blanket instead of the fluid-filled blanket to rewarm postoperative patients. The nurse implements this change for his or her own patients and monitors those patients' rewarming times, frequency of cardiac dysrhythmias, cost, and electrolyte balance. The nurse finds that rewarming times are shorter, dysrhythmias are less frequent, electrolyte imbalances are reduced, and the cost of care is less. As a result of this change, this nurse's idea becomes a hospital-wide protocol. This nurse then disseminates his or her findings in a publication and is invited to address critical care nurses at a regional conference. The nurse's findings are validated at other institutions, and eventually a state-of-the-art postoperative rewarming standard of care is accepted. This is an example of how one idea, which is acted on and followed through by nurses, can generate a significant difference for patients and cost savings for the institutions.

Perhaps more nurses need to advocate "killing sacred cows," not always sticking to a plan, and an "if it ain't broke, break it" philosophy. Such "radical" thinking allows more participation in developing a vision that is exciting, creating a future that is challenging, and creating new opportunities.

Consider the following: "In ten years all current knowledge and accepted practice will be obsolete . . . the life span of new technology [will be] decreased to 18 months . . . 20 times as many people will work at home, and ... three-fourths of [all] U.S. families will have two paychecks" (Kriegal & Palter, 1991, p. xviii). Certainly these predictions are startling, but because trends like these will have a major impact on the future, they validate why leaders, organizations, and groups need to attend to trends, engage in continuous change, and work to create a preferred future.

General Predictions about the Future

It is difficult not to be slightly pessimistic when considering some of the predictions about the future: global warming with its concurrent ecological collapse, nuclear or biological warfare, growing terrorism, increased violence, economic demise, and infectious diseases that are resistant to antibiotic therapy. However, such predictions also can serve to challenge us to plan proactively to minimize these possibilities and their negative effects, as well as to promote enthusiasm about countering these trends, for example, by developing superantibiotics, connecting to alien civilizations, increasing the quality of life and life span, benefiting from our ability to map all 80,000 genes in human DNA, strengthening the total world infrastructure, and using solar power.

> *"If there is no struggle, there is no progress."*
> —Frederick Douglass

Advancements in consumer electronics will assist in greater communication; easier access to services; at-home jobs; less time traveling in cars, trains, and planes; increased leisure time; and new education avenues. Just for a moment, think about this possibility: all roads and cars are removed from the earth, the old roads are made into moving sidewalks where one steps on and with a handheld apparatus controls the direction and speed of one's trip. Just think of the decrease in trauma that would result if there were no cars to have accidents with other vehicles, pedestrians, and animals. The current reality is that most people still have cars, and traffic jams and accidents still exist. However, we can still envision a preferred future in which energy is conserved and more travelers use superfast rail systems and suborbital space travel. Changes such as these will affect global trade, influence how people interact with one another and how they spend their time, and possibly assist people in living a more productive life.

In addition to changes such as these, dramatic changes in family structures and population demographics will continue to occur. The family will no longer be the primary social unit. Today 40 percent of American children have no father living in their home, and this trend is expected to continue (McRae, 1994). The U.S. population currently makes up 4.7 percent of the world population, but it will make up only 4 percent of the world population in 25 years. Thus America is not growing in population size the way many other countries are growing. There will be fewer young people in America, and the United States will have less of a voice regarding national and global issues. As the U.S. society ages (12.6 percent of the population is older than 65 years in 1998; 21.5 percent are predicted to be older than 65 years in 2030; and 27 percent of the population will be older than 65 years in 2050), the retirement age is predicted to increase to 70 years in 2025 (Molitor, 1998, p. 55). Because of the increase in the elderly population and the decrease in the younger population, the United States may give more priority to issues affecting the old versus those issues influencing the young. Diversity of the U.S. population will continue until fewer than 50 percent of U.S. citizens are from European descent in 2100 (Molitor, 1998, pp. 55–56). With the increased number of retirees and decreased number of workers, the Social Security system is expected to be insolvent in 2030, if not sooner. Medicare also is expected to be nearly insolvent by 2008, so new approaches to provide healthcare to the elderly, poor, and underserved will need to be created. Ethical considerations for caring for the elderly, critically ill individuals with multiple organ disease, the disabled, and those found to have genetic defects also will be more prevalent and force us to explore new alternatives to providing care for the very ill and dying.

Predictions about the Future of Healthcare

Healthcare costs were approximately $1 trillion in 1996; they are expected to be $1.4 trillion in 2000 (Molitor, 1998). It is no wonder, then, that cost is a major issue in healthcare today. However, as capitated financial arrangements are established and cost issues are addressed, the issue of quality of healthcare also is receiving long-awaited attention. This emphasis on the quality of services provided at a reasonable cost has many benefits, such as more educated consumers, certification for healthcare providers, choice of healthcare provider (e.g., nurse practitioner or nurse midwife, as well as physician), more health partnerships, more independence for nurse and other nonphysician providers, telehealth, an outcomes-driven system, and of course, improved care for patients, families, and communities. The emphasis on quality and on the measurement of outcomes will require all healthcare professionals to be accountable and responsible for providing competent interventions that generate positive patient outcomes. In addition, educators of healthcare providers will need to be role models who practice in their given field while they maintain expertise in their teaching roles.

Healthcare will focus increasingly on the prevention of illness and the promotion of health, and more care will be provided in short-stay units, urgent-care centers, subacute facilities, and homes. Healthcare will move from isolated, free-standing agencies to integrated networks that focus not only on primary or tertiary care but on the entire continuum of healthcare delivery. In other words, hospitals and acute-care centers will continue to develop affiliations with other hospitals, rehabilitation centers, subacute-care facilities, community centers, long-term care facilities, and laboratories, as well as develop satellite centers in the community to provide primary and secondary care to neighborhoods. Hospitals will no longer deal merely with health restoration but with health promotion and maintenance as well. To be effective in the future, healthcare systems will need to "embrace a mission of community service" (Rohrer, 1998, p. 400) and be an integral part of the community in which they exist.

Bezold and Mayer (1996) suggest the following as possibilities in the future of healthcare: microrobots that circulate through the vascular system slowing the aging process and repairing the body of disease, dream therapy that allows dreaming via virtual reality techniques to create healthier people, and some type of communication system that allows for interaction between one's consciousness and cells. New techniques in diagnostic technology and genetic research are expected to move us from a "diagnose and treat" scenario (once symptoms are manifested) to a "predict and manage prophylactically" scenario (even before symptoms are evident).

Computerization will continue to allow all providers to access the patient's record, regardless of location, and patients/consumers themselves will be able to access their records freely. Multidisciplinary teams involving physicians, nurses, social workers, physical therapists, psychologists, occupational therapists, and other providers we cannot even envision today will follow evidence-based protocols to deliver quality care to patients, and they will be delivering that care in the patient's home or community, including schools, malls, workplaces, satellite health centers, and other access points. These differences between the current healthcare delivery system and what integrated delivery systems (IDSs) of the future will be like are summarized in Table 8–2.

Predictions about the Future of Nursing

As stated earlier, nurses must become involved in predicting the future; in fact, nurses must be involved in creating a preferred future. If we agree with Bennis (1989, p. 191) that "chaos is a source of energy and it is the beginning not the end" and if we agree that the healthcare system is in chaos, then now is the time for nurses to create the future that will benefit patients and communities and that will best utilize all that nursing has to offer. Many elements of the chaos in healthcare, such as downsizing of healthcare institutions, changing from an illness to a wellness perspective, moving

Table 8–2 *Characteristics of the Past/Traditional and Future Healthcare Systems*

Past/Traditional Healthcare System	Future Healthcare System
Episodic, fragmented	Continuous, coordinated
Individualized plan of care	Critical pathways
Sickness-focused	Health promotion- and prevention-focused
Insurance coverage	Managed care organizations
Inpatient care	Ambulatory and community-based care
Hospital as profit center	Hospital as cost center
Specialist physicians	Primary care practitioners
Independent solo physicians	Multispecialty group practice
Physician-dominated care	Nonphysician care providers
Fee-for-service payments	Predetermined capitated fee payments
Heavily regulated environment	Increasingly competitive environment
Provider-oriented	Consumer-oriented
Presumption of high quality	Documented quality

Source: Adapted from Buerhaus, P. (1998). Creating a new place in a competitive market: The value of nursing care. In E.C. Hein (Ed.), *Contemporary leadership behavior: Selected readings* (5th ed.) (p. 424). Philadelphia: Lippincott.

from private physician–dominated providers to multidisciplinary systems, and the use of capitated payment systems, all have significance for nursing. In addition, many demographic changes, such as the increasing elderly population, more fatherless families, more ethnic diversity, more homelessness, and more underprivileged people needing healthcare in their communities, provide increased opportunities for more autonomous nursing practice.

The nursing workforce itself needs more baccalaureate- and master's-prepared nurses who practice autonomously, use evidence-based nursing interventions that generate positive patient outcomes, are respected as the experts in certain areas of patient care, develop health policy, and collaborate fully with a multidisciplinary healthcare team. Both registered nurses (RNs) and advanced practice nurses (APNs) *must* be accountable for patient outcomes and eliminate old ways of thinking, such as "a nurse reports to the physician and merely needs to notify the physician about a change or document in the patient record a finding about a patient." Instead, if we are to create a preferred future for nursing, nurses must be responsible in following through via appropriate mechanisms in identifying a problem, concern, or anything a nurse deems out of the ordinary enough to notify a physician about, until the patient outcome is realized. The future of the profession depends on nurses' following through, taking responsibility, and documenting the outcomes of their research-based interventions. Only then will we truly be able to "sit at the table" with our colleagues from other healthcare disciplines and be recognized for contributing significantly to quality and cost-effective care.

High technology, including patient monitoring systems, computerized medication administration, interactive computer communication, and computerized patient data storage, is a good example of how nursing can benefit from change. Technological advances such as those just mentioned maximize the potential for nurses to spend more time with patients, allow more independent clinical judgments, provide immediate ability to communicate with other members of the healthcare team, and help nurses manage patient data for quick retrieval when analyzing patient outcomes. Technology, therefore, is not an enemy but an ally because it helps nurses be more autonomous.

The passing of the Balanced Budget Act of 1997, mandating direct payment to nurse practitioners, has had a huge impact on the future of advanced practice nursing. However, nursing leaders must be certain to collaborate with the Medicare Commission to develop healthcare policy that allows this third-party payment to continue and be expanded. In fact, to shape the preferred future for nursing, all nurses should be involved with developing health policy, networking with legislators and political groups, and spearheading changes in the delivery of health education and healthcare to consumers. Such action will enable nurses to influence necessary changes in healthcare, and it also will improve the profession's image as a competent and powerful contributor to the health of the American people.

No longer can nurses focus solely on their particular unit or their own specialty area. Today's nurses cannot expect to work for the same employer throughout their career, nor can they expect to do the same thing in nursing throughout their career. They must therefore be aware of the larger arena of healthcare, continue their education, and remain flexible. Nurses also will do well to focus on measuring nursing outcomes, being attuned to cost effectiveness, ensuring high-quality nursing interventions, being a part of ethical debates, providing access to healthcare to all, working collaboratively with one another and with other healthcare professionals, increasing our educational preparation standards, and being a vital voice in healthcare policy making.

> *"Quality is never an accident; it is always the result of intelligent effort."*
> —John Ruskin

Nurses must take responsibility for shaping the future of the nursing profession, as well as for shaping their own careers. By studying patterns of change, being aware of important trends in one's specific area of nursing, keeping abreast of general healthcare literature, and talking to others involved in healthcare, nurses will be more able to deal with the unexpected that the future is bound to bring.

It is important to realize that no single individual can decide what the future will be. However, nurses can shape that future by being more cognizant of possibilities and more open to trying new and radical changes. We cannot sit back passively and merely accept everything the future hands us; instead, we must create the preferred future of nursing. But how can we do that? Some of the following strategies may help nurses become more effective decision makers and influencers regarding healthcare issues in the next century.

EDUCATIONAL PREPARATION FOR NURSES

The American Association of Colleges of Nursing's (1997) position statement, *A Vision of Baccalaureate and Graduate Nursing Education,* states that it is the responsibility of nursing educators along with nurse executives and clinicians in practice settings to shape practice and not merely respond to changes. Nursing education must prepare practitioners who have the ability to participate as full partners in healthcare delivery and shape health policy. Therefore, nurses must have a minimum of a baccalaureate degree for entry into professional practice. Nursing curricula should emphasize primary care, patient education, health promotion, rehabilitation, self-care, and alternative methods of healing, while not eliminating or minimizing too drastically the focus on acute and tertiary care (American Association of Colleges of Nursing, 1997, p. 2). All curricula should include, at appropriate levels, case management, healthcare policy, research, quality indicators, outcome measures, financial management, legislative advocacy, trends toward privatization, and management of data. The notion of lifelong learning for all nurses to maintain competency also must be addressed, perhaps in a mandatory continuing education or through certification, either of which could be required for relicensure.

WORKFORCE, LICENSURE, AND REGULATION

The PEW Commission on Nursing (Donaho, 1997) recommended a number of changes that can assist the nursing profession in creating a preferred future. These workforce, licensure, and regulation issues include the following:

- *Standardizing regulatory terms:* Nurses must use consistent terminology to designate who they are, RN, APN, or LPN.
- *Standardizing entry into practice requirements:* Nurses must address the various levels of entry and also focus on competence with assessment.
- *Removing barriers to the full use of competent professionals:* Nurses must evaluate how nurses are deemed competent throughout their careers; merely holding a basic license cannot ensure competence to work in every area of nursing because nursing practice is extremely specialized.
- *Redesigning the state board structure and function:* Nurses must enable more focus on healthcare policy, role definition, and protocol development. Changing the process from one in which board members and chair are appointed by the state governor to a process in which such individuals are elected (via the state nurses' association or some other peer group) would allow broader involvement and representation.
- *Informing the public:* Nurses must communicate their credentials and competencies to the consumer so that the public is aware of the RN and APN role in the practice arena.
- *Collecting data on the workforce:* The nursing workforce must be studied to ensure wise distribution and appropriate mix of competencies at the various levels of practice.
- *Ensuring the competence of practitioners:* Nurses must develop an ongoing certification process for all practitioners at the RN and APN levels.
- *Reforming the professional disciplinary process:* Nurses must publicize who is practicing unsafely.
- *Evaluating regulatory effectiveness:* State boards of nursing must evaluate their effectiveness and efficiency.
- *Understanding the organizational context of health professions regulation:* Nurses must streamline the number of regulatory bodies that govern nursing practice.

Essentially, nurses must define exactly what nursing does and communicate it to the public so that consumers will be able to understand the role of the RN and APN.

Expansion of the Role of the Nurse

Porter-O'Grady (1997a) recommends that nurses expand their roles to work as consultants to the public, patient or professional specialty groups, healthcare equipment or pharmaceutical corporations, day-care centers, or any group interested in health. This exemplary role model of an entrepreneur in nursing says that "the skills of the consultant, grounded in practice and framed by the discipline of nursing" (p. 28), more than adequately prepare the nurse to take on the expanding demand of the consultant's role. The future will open the consultant role to more baccalaureate- and master's-prepared nurses who have "sound clinical roots and the insight of 'having been there'" (Porter-O'Grady, 1997a, p. 28), and this will help increase the public's knowledge of what nurses actually do.

MEMBERSHIP AND PARTICIPATION IN PROFESSIONAL NURSING ORGANIZATIONS

All nurses should be involved in a professional nursing organization that is actively working to create a preferred future for the profession. Sigma Theta Tau International's (STTI's) 1997–1999 biennium theme, for example, was "Avenues to the Future," a theme centered around creating collaborative partnerships and refocusing the public's image of nursing. STTI and other organizations (e.g., the American Association of Critical Care Nurses and the Emergency Nurses Association) have committed to creating a positive future by offering leadership institutes, teaching members how to network with each other more through the Internet or newsletters, and offering recognition through awards and citations as a way to motivate nurses to work at their highest possible level. Whether one is working at the local or chapter level as a committee member or officer, serving on a board of directors, working on an international committee, or reviewing manuscripts for an organization's journal, one is working to advance the future of nursing and helping shape that future.

SIGNIFICANCE OF NURSING RESEARCH

For a preferred future, nurses must develop patient care protocols that are evidence-based. Research must be conducted to determine the extent to which caregivers adhere to these protocols, the cost-effectiveness of using them, and the positive and negative (e.g., complications) patient outcomes generated when such protocols are used. Nurses should be able to autonomously change protocols that affect nursing care of patients.

Nurses must study the effectiveness of what we do and participate in multidisciplinary research, providing leadership for the nursing aspect of such research. We must continue to study the healthcare practices of various groups and then broaden this focus to study patients' responses to specific interventions. The time has come for nurses to measure the effect of nursing care and not merely describe problems that exist in healthcare. Dissemination of results should be done in publications and presentations, including those that are multidisciplinary in nature, and the commitment to using research results as a basis for practice and conducting research must be integral to every nurse's ongoing practice.

OUTCOMES OF NURSING INTERVENTIONS

Nurses can improve quality outcomes and initiate actions to measure and track indicators of nursing quality. If we do not develop outcome variables that reflect nurses' actions, our contributions will be less valued (Buerhaus, 1998, p. 428). In 1966 Donabedian constructed three categories of interdependent quality determinants: structure (e.g., facilities, equipment, staff, and other resources through which services are provided); process (e.g., characteristics of service delivery that create value for the patient, such as safety, availability, and appropriateness); and outcomes (e.g., results of the actions). Quality is measured by the outcomes achieved, a process referred to (in the corporate arena) as total quality management (TQM) or continuous quality improvement (CQI). Nurses should implement an outcomes-based quality process for each nursing intervention performed so that their contributions to patient care are documented.

Arrington and Kurz (1995, p. 290) recommend that all quality-improvement programs include four essential areas to promote continued growth of indicator measurement: "development of knowledge specifically supportive of improvement efforts; use of strategic leadership to leverage organizational quality improvement efforts by cultivating a shared sense of purpose and focus, encouraging improved performance, and promoting organizational learning; mastery of methods and tools that accelerate improved performance; and demonstration of ever-increasing ability to develop new knowledge and apply it to improving the processes of daily work." Nurses can enhance their focus on quality by attending to these four areas in their efforts to improve care and create a preferred future.

The Nursing Minimum Data Set Committees of the American Nurses Association and the American Organization of Nurse Executives have been making great strides in establishing a universal taxonomy of nursing minimum data. These nursing data should be included in outcomes research (Simpson, 1997), particularly outcomes that relate to clinical, economic, and humanistic dimensions, such as symptom relief, functional capacity, cost, resource use, and complications.

To maximize the contributions of nursing, it is mandatory for nurses to participate in outcome measurements because the shift in healthcare from evaluating only cost variables to determining both cost and quality perspectives will continue. Wouldn't it be beneficial for nursing if consumer evaluation identified nursing interventions as a part of what made them decide to use a specific agency, hospital, or service provider?

Leaders create bridges—interconnections between people that empower them and that change their focus from merely "doing their jobs" to having a larger purpose. Leaders must be integrators—people who can see beyond the differences among various members of the group or team and use these divergent talents and perspectives to benefit the group. They must be diplomats—people who can help people get past their conflicts with one another and facilitate their working together. Leaders must be "cross-fertilizers"—individuals who bring the best out of each group or individual and allow that to be shared with the entire team. And they must be deep thinkers—those who can see all kinds of possibilities even when no progress seems to be being made (Kanter, 1996). In essence, leaders foster collaboration among individuals and keep lines of communication open between all group members.

> *"You don't have to be brilliant to be a good leader. But you do have to understand other people—how they feel, what makes them tick, and the best way to influence them."*
>
> —John Luther

As noted earlier, the chaotic world of today needs more than just a few leaders at the top. Leadership is not a position but a process and a role that everyone can and must assume at some point in time. Staub (1996) suggests we look for leaders at all levels of society and organizations through "fuzzy logic," an approach of "approximations" (p. xv). An example of fuzzy logic and approximations is the difference between a regular light switch, which turns a light on or off, and a dimmer switch, which allows a light to vary in degrees of brightness. According to Staub (1996, p. xv), the dimmer switch, or fuzzy logic, "allows for a greater range of response and therefore flexibility to the requirements of the environment. . . . So too, in real life, [where] the range of options can be extended to many more iterations between the two fixed positions of off or on, right or wrong, black or white. In approaching the challenge of our complex world, it is important to remember that while white matters and black matters, where it really counts is in gray matter(s)."

In essence, everyone has something to offer; there is a place on the team where each person can make important contributions. Perhaps if the strengths of individuals were appreciated and they were empowered, members of a team would develop the self-confidence to do their very best and make significant contributions to shaping a preferred future. This attitude of people working hard and

> *"The reward of a thing well done, it to have done it."*
> —Ralph Waldo Emerson

feeling good about themselves, and having their contributions go a long way in accomplishing a once seemingly hopeless task or vision, is the essence of collaboration.

Partnering implies teamwork, with every member being equal and all connecting horizontally, not vertically, or via a web structure (Helgesen, 1990). Using principles of partnership such as equity, accountability, and ownership, each member contributes a unique set of talents to achieve the common goal, such as quality patient care. Everything the partners do is patient-focused, and no one tells another partner what to do or when to do it. Indeed, the new healthcare system will not support this type of authoritative behavior; instead, it will expect each person to own his or her part and do his or her job with excellence (Porter-O'Grady, 1997b). Such a paradigm supports collaboration, dialog, patient participation, freedom of expression, and empowerment (Rost, 1993), all of which are crucial to success.

Instead of complaining about being the only ones at the bedside continuously—24 hours around the clock in hospitals, daily at homes, and weekly in clinics—nurses should take pride in the responsibility they have to monitor patients and provide health surveillance in primary care settings and the community. Instead of seeing ourselves as mere coordinators or implementers of tasks ordered by others, we should take pride in the leadership we provide as case managers and the way we are the "glue" that holds it all together. This is what nurses do, and it is our unique contribution to the healthcare team. With the increase in equal partnering, nursing has a new frontier to pursue and new roles to assume.

Finally, the preferred future for nursing incorporates nurses working as independent providers rather than being employees of a healthcare agency. For example, patients who need education about their health may be served by a nurse entrepreneur who has been called on by a multidisciplinary team, the patient, or another nurse. Or a healthcare agency that has a large population of new diabetic patients might contract with a nurse who is specialized in diabetes to do the teaching for these patients. Nurses now have many opportunities to work as independent providers, and such opportunities are expected to increase in the future. By partnering and networking with other healthcare workers and by marketing one's abilities, nurses will be recognized as experts, and their talents will be used appropriately.

Characteristics of Nurse Leaders Needed to Create a Preferred Future for Nursing

Leaders of tomorrow must be transformational ones—people who can propel a vision, empower followers to work enthusiastically to realize a vision, meet change "head-on" and grow from it, explore conflict to ensure people are thinking in different ways, and keep harmful stress at a minimum for themselves and the organization. They must be designers, teachers, and stewards (Senge, 1990): *designers* assist in developing the vision; *teachers* help followers develop the skills and gain the knowledge to work toward making the vision a reality; and *stewards* act as spokespersons for the group, keep the group focused on the vision, and facilitate the long-term growth of all followers.

> *"What makes a leader—intelligence, integrity, imagination, skill: in brief, statecraft? Not at all. It is the fact that the man has a following."*
>
> —Gerald W. Johnson (American Journalist, 1890–1980)

Leaders have ideas about what the future can bring and what it could be like, but they do not just sit around and wait for things to happen. Leaders for the future take action, engage in self-evaluation, seek feedback from colleagues, set goals and periodically evaluate progress in meeting them, advance their own knowledge, and try new things (Valiga, 1994). Being able to envision the future separates leaders from others.

Accepting the challenge of leading is a decision each of us must make. When we accept that challenge, we may be more successful in shaping a preferred future if we incorporate the following perspectives (Bennis, 1989, pp. 192–199):

- Manage the dream . . . take the vision to reality.
- Embrace error . . . never be afraid to fail or to admit it.
- Encourage reflective back talk . . . have someone you trust serve as a sounding board for your ideas.

- Encourage dissent . . . play the role of devil's advocate and encourage others to do the same.
- Possess the "Nobel" (p. 196) . . . be optimistic, have hope, and have faith.
- Understand the "Pygmalion effect" (p. 197) . . . how you treat followers will determine how followers perform.
- Develop the "Gretzky factor" (p. 199) . . . know where the hockey puck will be, not just where it is.
- See the long view . . . be forward looking and have a broad perspective.
- Understand the stakeholder's symmetry . . . balance everyone's competing claims in the group.
- Create strategic alliances and partnerships . . . the dream cannot be accomplished alone.

The next generation of leaders—those who will create the preferred future for nursing—will need "a broad education, boundless curiosity and enthusiasm, belief in people and teamwork, willingness to take risks, devotion to long-term growth rather than short-term profit, commitment to excellence, readiness, virtue, and vision" (Bennis, 1989, p. 202).

Individuals must accept the challenge of leadership. They also may be more successful in shaping a preferred future if they incorporate another set of guidelines (Kouzes & Posner, 1995, p. 99):

- Do not wait.
- Have credibility . . . be honest, be an inspiration, maintain competence, and be forward-looking.
- Have your head in the clouds but your feet on the ground . . . always be thinking of possibilities but also stay grounded in reality.

> "Never give up your credibility by saying, 'This may be a dumb question, but . . .'"
> —Elizabeth Tegues

- Share values.
- Accept that you cannot do it alone.
- Remember that leadership is everyone's business.

As long as one has a vision, articulates it clearly, enlists others to help make it reality, is aware of factors that influence it, and is able to keep the vision on course, one really is a leader and is shaping a preferred future. It is much more exciting to help determine what the future will be than to merely react to it as it happens around us. True wisdom and true leadership come from learning from the past, enjoying and growing in the present, preparing for the future, and creating the future.

CONCLUSION

The role of the nurse is expanding and will continue to expand. In light of this, all nurses must decide how much and in what directions we want that role to continue to expand and then plan strategies to make it happen. It would seem that all nurses can embrace the vision of providing quality healthcare to anyone in need. What we need to do now is work collaboratively to make this vision a reality. No longer can we merely follow the directions of others; we must continue to engage in critical thinking and effectively communicate with our equal partners on the healthcare team to determine the best actions for care that is of the highest quality.

Leadership must be everybody's business, and every nurse must take a part in standing up for a cause, bridging a gap, networking with others, and doing what needs to be done to move our profession forward toward *the future we want*. Apathy, doing only what is written in one's job description, retorting "I am only a nurse" or "That is not my job," failing to continue to learn, letting others make decisions for us, or continuing to assume a subservient role will not serve us well in the evolving healthcare system, and it will not help us create a preferred future for nursing.

Critical Thinking 8–1

Critical Thinking Exercises

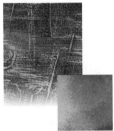

Imagine that it is the year 2005 and you are about to be interviewed by
an international nursing journal about the significant difference you
have made to the nursing profession. What would you talk about? What significant differences have
you made? How will you respond when the interviewer asks what you plan to do in the next 5 years to
continue to make a difference?

_____

_____

Draw a picture of your vision of the role of the nurse in your current area of employment for the future.
What could you do to make this vision a reality? Share your ideas with your nurse manager or colleagues.

_____

_____

Identify four positive and four negative events related to your nursing career or your experiences as a
nursing student that you have experienced in the past. Describe why each may have happened. Review
the positive ones and determine a pattern, and review the negative ones to see if a pattern emerges
there. What can you learn from this analysis that could help you shape your own professional future?

_____

_____

Given the predictions about the future in general, the future of healthcare, and the future of nursing,
what kinds of nurse leaders will the profession need to shape a preferred future? Are these same
qualities needed today? Why or why not?

_____

_____

Informally interview a variety of people (e.g., children, an elderly person, a healthcare provider, nurse colleagues, a new college graduate) about the future of our society, our world, the healthcare system, and nursing. Ask them what they think things will be like in the year 2010 and beyond. Also ask them what they think we need to do now to achieve the positive things they envision and avoid the negative things they envision. Are the views of nurses different from those of other groups?

References

Arrington, B., & Kurz, R. (1995). Quality management and improvement. In W.J. Duncan, P. Ginter, & L.E. Swayne (Eds.), *Handbook of healthcare management* (pp. 285–310). Malden, MA: Blackwell Business.

American Association of Colleges of Nursing. (1997). *AACN position statement: A vision of baccalaureate and graduate nursing education.* Washington, D.C.: American Association of Colleges of Nursing.

Bennis, W. (1989). *On becoming a leader.* Reading, MA: Addison-Wesley.

Bezold, C. (1996). Your health in 2010: Four scenarios. *The Futurist 30*(5), 35–39.

Bezold, C., & Mayer, E. (Eds.). (1996). *Future care responding to the demand for change.* New York: Faulkner & Gray.

Buerhaus, P. (1998). Creating a new place in a competitive market: The value of nursing care. In E.C. Hein (Ed.), *Contemporary leadership behavior: Selected readings* (5th ed.) (pp. 422–431). Philadelphia: Lippincott.

Donabedian, A. (1966). Evaluating the quality of medical care. *Milbank Memorial Fund Quarterly 44*(3), 166–203.

Donaho, B. (1997). The PEW Commission report: Nursing's challenge to address it. *ANNA Journal 2*, 507–514.

Helgesen, S. (1990). *The female advantage: Women's ways of leadership.* New York: Doubleday Currency.

Kanter, R. (1996). World class leaders. In F. Hesselbein, M. Goldsmith, & R. Beckhard (Eds.), *The leader of the future* (pp. 89–98). San Francisco: Jossey-Bass.

Kouzes, J., & Posner, B. (1995). *The leadership challenge: How to keep getting extraordinary things done in organizations* (2nd ed.). San Francisco: Jossey-Bass.

Kriegal, R., & Palter, L. (1991). *If it ain't broke, break it.* New York: Warner Books.

McRae, H. (1994). *2020 vision: Power, culture, prosperity.* Cambridge, MA: Harvard Business School Press.

Minkin, B. (1995). *Future in sight.* New York: Macmillan.

Molitor, G. (1998). Trends and forecasts for the new millennium. *The Futurist 32*(6), 53–59.

Naisbitt, J., & Auburdeen, P. (1990). *Megatrends 2000: Ten new directions for the 1990s.* New York: W. Morrow.

Nanus, B. (1992). *Visionary leadership: Creating a compelling sense of direction for your organization.* San Francisco: Jossey-Bass.

Porter-O'Grady, T. (1997a). The private practice of nursing entrepreneurialism. *Nursing Administration Quarterly 22*(1), 23–29.

Porter-O'Grady, T. (1997b). Over the horizon: The future and the advanced practice nurse. *Nursing Administration Quarterly 21*(4), 1–11.

Rohrer, J. (1998). Designing effective healthcare organizations for the future. In W.J. Duncan, P.M. Ginter, & L.E. Swayne (Eds.), *Handbook of healthcare management* (pp. 399–432). Malden, MA: Blackwell Business.

Rost, J. (1993). *Leadership for the 21st century.* Westport, CT: Praeger.

Senge, P. (1990). *The fifth discipline: The art and practice of the learning organization.* New York: Doubleday.

Simpson, R. (1997). Including nursing in medical outcomes research. *Nursing Management 28,* 26–27.

Staub, R. (1996). *The heart of leadership: Twelve practices of courageous leaders.* Provo, UT: Executive Excellence.

Toffler, A. (1990). *Powershift.* New York: Bantam.

Valiga, T. (1994). Leadership for the future. *Holistic Nursing Practice 9*(1), 83–90.

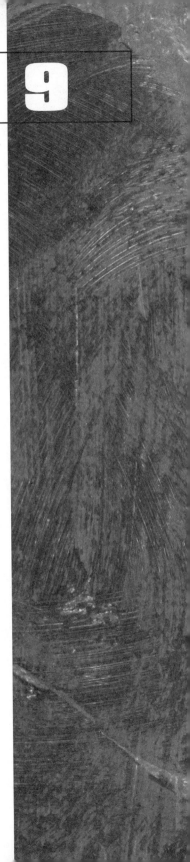

CHAPTER **9**

Developing as a Leader throughout One's Career

Developing as a Leader throughout One's Career

Learning Objectives

☐ Describe ways in which individuals can develop as leaders.

☐ Describe the characteristics of an environment that facilitates the development of leadership skills in self and others.

☐ Relate the concept of empowerment to the development of leaders.

☐ Analyze the process of mentoring as it relates to the development of leaders.

☐ Propose a personal plan for leadership development that attends to empowerment, mentoring, role modeling, networking, self-assessment, and continued renewal.

INTRODUCTION

Although one of the early leadership theories, the Great Man Theory, espoused that leaders were individuals who had been born into the "right" family at the "right" time, this theory has been challenged over the years as being far from useful in understanding the multifaceted nature of leadership. Indeed, there is now widespread agreement that leaders are made, not born. But the question remains as to how an individual can be "made" into a leader.

Individuals who are acknowledged as leaders do not simply declare that they will be leaders and expect that others will accept such a declaration. Instead, individuals who are acknowledged as leaders often are nurtured and guided by others, seek and function in environments that encourage leadership behavior, "test" the role, and study others who have been leaders.

Thus, the development of oneself as a leader is a purposeful process that is enhanced by guidance and support from others. But what are the ways in which one can develop leadership skills? This chapter explores numerous approaches to leadership development, and several of the strategies that have particular relevance for nurses are examined in depth.

General Approaches to Leadership Development

Emergence as a leader is a developmental learning process in which capacities, insights, and skills gained through one experience or at one level serve as the basis for further growth; thus, leaders go through stages in their development. It also is generally acknowledged that one learns to be a leader by serving as a leader: merely talking about being a leader or observing others in that role does not make one a leader. One is a leader when he or she exercises leadership.

Based on one's past performance or promise of future performance, one often is expected to provide leadership to a group. As a person has success in that role, more and more leadership is expected of that individual; thus one may continually be "promoted" to higher levels of leadership responsibility.

Finally, leadership development is a lifelong process. As nurses progress throughout their careers, they will face new challenges. The need for change will always exist, and groups will need leaders to help them weather the forces of change. Conflict will also always exist, particularly as resources become more scarce and new healthcare workers challenge traditional roles; groups will need leaders to help them manage those conflicts. New visions will continually need to be articulated as previous visions are realized or changing societal expectations demand new directions; groups will need leaders to help them see and realize those new visions. As the circumstances of our lives are constantly altered, our leadership skills also need to be refined, renewed, and further developed.

LECTURE AND DISCUSSION: FORMAL COURSE WORK

Perhaps one of the most common and easiest ways to develop leadership skills is through participation in lectures, discussions, or formal course work on leadership. Such experiences provide information about the phenomenon, facilitate a "formal" examination of individuals who have demonstrated leadership in the past or in contemporary society, and stimulate thinking about the nature of leadership and followership. Participation in an effective discussion group also provides experience in working with others to reach decisions and helps one develop an awareness of the need for more than single, simple answers to complex problems.

In addition to isolated or clusters of lectures and discussions about leadership, many universities have instituted programs that focus on leadership. The University of Richmond (Virginia) offered the first baccalaureate program in leadership in 1992, and Chapman University (California) and Fort Hays State University (Kansas) have since added their own majors in this field. The University of Denver's "Pioneer Leadership Program" (Reisberg, 1998) combines classroom instruction with adventure-based outings as a way to develop leadership abilities, and it leads to a minor in leadership studies. At least eight institutions now offer minors in leadership studies, and a source book of courses and programs in leadership (Schwartz, 1998) has been developed to document the growth of such opportunities.

In 1992 the National Student Nurses Association (NSNA) developed an independent study module that was intended to serve as a model for schools to involve students as active participants in learning about leadership, developing leadership skills, and enhancing professional socialization. Through individualized learning contracts with faculty members, students use their experiences as the chairperson of a local Student Nurses Association (SNA) chapter or committee to study their own leadership style, gain confidence when leading groups, appreciate the many facets of group decision making, and understand the legislative process.

Finally, many nursing education programs have credit-bearing courses or noncredit workshops that deal with leadership and its development. Individuals wanting to learn more about this complex concept and the effective exercise of leadership, particularly in nursing and healthcare, may benefit from enrolling in such courses. However, it would be wise to study the course offering carefully before enrolling to be certain that it does indeed focus on leadership rather than on management.

ROLE-PLAYING AND SIMULATION

Although it often makes people uncomfortable, participation in role-playing or simulation exercises is an excellent way to develop leadership skills. By being expected to play the role of leader, one must be articulate, forward-thinking, creative, able to manage conflict and resolve differences among group members, acknowledge and build on the strengths of followers, and help the group move forward. Role-playing also can serve as a "diagnostic technique," through which one's strengths and areas needing improvement become apparent. For example, it will be evident if the individual playing the role of leader cannot articulate a vision clearly; the individual will then know that this is a particular skill needing more development.

Role-playing and simulation also can serve as a way to "test" various solutions to problems before actually being in the problem situation. For example, a group might construct a scenario in which one of their members plays the passive "sheep" follower role (Kelley, 1992) and the leader must figure out ways to help that follower become more effective. Knowing that reality often presents leaders with many "sheep" followers, being able to address this situation through role-playing gives leaders an opportunity to generate a number of approaches to dealing with such a situation before finding themselves actually faced with it. In addition, this kind of experience also provides other participants with an opportunity for vicarious learning in which they have observed which strategies were successful and which were not.

SENSITIVITY TRAINING

Participation in sensitivity training sessions that are led by expert facilitators provides participants with an opportunity to focus on openness, how hostilities and defensiveness may be exhibited within a group, and one's personal feelings, perceptions, and biases. It also increases one's sensitivity to others' needs and helps one appreciate the significance of shared decision making. Finally, such sessions also assist group members to reflect on the inner workings or processes of the group itself: who assumed what kinds of roles, who emerged as the leader, who was most effective in moving the group forward and why, and so on. Such insights are invaluable for those who will provide leadership in their work settings, professional associations, or communities.

> *"There's nothing wrong with a pleasant, good natured approach to people and problems—in fact, there's none better. The strange thing is that we so often forget to use it."*
> —Dwight Eisenhower

ROLE MODELING

Effective leadership skills can be developed by carefully observing individuals who are successful as leaders. By studying what such people do, how they communicate, how they motivate followers to "join in the cause," their level of energy and personal investment, their ability to keep the group focused on the vision despite conflicts and challenges along the way, and how their careers have evolved can be extremely helpful to the novice leader.

Role modeling occurs whether or not it is planned or purposeful. In other words, many of us pattern ourselves after others, even though we may not be aware of such unconscious "decisions," and we may find that we have adapted the negative or nonhelpful behaviors exhibited by others, as well as the positive or helpful ones. Therefore, role modeling is much more effective when it is done consciously and with deliberation.

Conscious or "formal" role modeling may be enhanced by attending professional conferences and conventions where one observes how participants conduct themselves, deal with "hot" issues that are open to debate, express opinions, and "connect" with members of the audience. It also can be achieved by being more observant during meetings one attends: who is typically able to convince the group that his or her point is the one that should be supported, and what does he or she do that makes him or her so convincing? Conscious role modeling can occur when one reads articles or editorials written by nurse leaders and reflects on their communication style, their willingness to address controversial topics publicly, and the fact that they use print media to convey a strongly held message or articulate a vision. Finally, it can be facilitated by reading biographies about leaders—in nursing or outside, contemporary or historical—and studying what they did and how they did it.

INSTITUTIONS AND FELLOWSHIPS

A more formalized approach to leadership development occurs through participation in institutes and fellowships. Such opportunities are announced in professional publications and are open to a wide variety of individuals.

In 1998, for example, the American Academy of Nursing and the American Nurses Foundation formed a partnership to develop an Institute for Nursing Leadership. The aim of this institute is to "build new leadership capacities through self-assessment, skill-building learning modules, and programs designed to connect nurses with mentors, sponsors and other . . . contacts" (Ferguson, 1998, p. 10). It is multifocused and relevant to nurses at all stages of their careers: fostering leadership skill building among under-graduate and graduate nursing students, fostering leadership competencies for nurses at early and emerging career points, facilitating mentoring and networking for nurses in their first managerial position, brokering access to leadership development programs (with executives outside their traditional work settings) for senior executive nurses, and enhancing connections with leaders in the field to maintain leadership capacity in the profession.

Sigma Theta Tau International, the Honor Society of Nursing, has as one of its major goals the development of leadership among its members. The ultimate purpose of focusing on leadership is to promote the discovery, dissemination, and utilization of knowledge to improve the health of individuals and communities worldwide. Through its workshops, programs, conferences, and International Leadership Institute, Sigma Theta Tau International serves to address the leadership development needs of nurses who are currently providing leadership at the local, regional, and international level and nurses who have the potential to provide such leadership. The goal of the Institute is to help nurses "be able to influence people, organizations and situations to bring about transforming change" (*Annual Report 1998,* 1999, p. 7).

The University of Kansas School of Nursing offers a summer leadership development institute for healthcare managers and executives, and the Colorado Alliance for Nursing has received a 3-year grant to develop a nursing leadership institute for nurses from medically underserved areas to help them function effectively in the evolving healthcare delivery system. The University of Chicago's International Center for Health Leadership Development conducts leadership development activities that help prepare leaders from communities, community health centers, and health professions education to build links and partnerships between communities and institutions; it helps individuals discover their leadership capabilities and helps them see that, in many ways, leadership is a function of the relationship between leaders and followers.

Another program in nursing that focuses on the development of leadership is the Leadership Initiative for Nursing Education Program, funded by the Helene Fuld Health Trust (New York). This initiative includes a 6-month fellowship and a 5-day leadership institute designed to enhance the leadership skills of both nurse educators and nursing students at the baccalaureate level and to promote closer relationships between nurse educators and employers, who seek to hire graduates prepared for the leadership challenges of the next century. The Center for Creative Leadership (North Carolina) is a well-established program that offers workshops, books, and other resources regarding leadership. Many more programs are designed to enhance leadership development.

ON-THE-JOB TRAINING

Perhaps the most effective way to develop as a successful leader is to use such skills "on the job." On-the-job training may include temporary job rotations to positions that require the use of new skills, assignment as an assistant or apprentice to someone in a leadership role, serving as the chair-elect of a committee, or participation in some leadership internship, such as those described previously or ones offered through one's employing agency. On-the-job training also may occur through a mentor relationship, a concept discussed in more depth later in this chapter.

> *"Knowing is not enough; we must apply. Willing is not enough; we must do."*
> —Goethe

SUMMARY

In essence, nurses who are seeking to develop or enhance their leadership skills and abilities would benefit from attending carefully to those in their work and professional environments (e.g., as potential role models) and considering becoming involved in some type of formal leadership training program. In selecting such a program, one should look for opportunities to examine the complex phenomenon of leadership in depth, be certain one chooses carefully between leadership development and management training programs, and choose a program that provides opportunities to actually experience the role of leader, receive thoughtful, critical feedback on one's performance in that role, and receive guidance in building on areas of strength and developing areas of weakness. Potential and effective nurse leaders also would be best served by practicing in an environment that facilitates their development as leaders.

Environments That Facilitate Leadership Development

Although aspiring leaders may not be in a position to create an environment that facilitates leadership development, they are likely to be in a position to choose to practice and participate in such environments. But what do such environments look like? What should nurses look for in such environments?

Much like those that promote creativity (see Chapter 5) and those that promote human development in general, environments that promote the development and enhancement of leadership skills and abilities are open, trusting, and dynamic. In such environments, individuals feel free to raise questions about what is being done, how it is being done, why it is being done in a particular way, and why it is being done at all. Not only is a questioning attitude accepted, it is encouraged and expected.

Environments that promote the development of leadership do not maintain the status quo and do not put individuals into "boxes," but they do encourage each person to reach his or her maximum potential. A spirit of competitiveness that constantly pushes members to achieve excellence may characterize the environment, but group members are not in competition with one another. Indeed, environments that facilitate the development of leadership recognize the strengths and talents of each member of the group, find ways to build on those strengths, and expect group members to guide, encourage, and support each other as they continue to grow. They are, in essence, environments in which leaders are allowed to emerge and followers are seen as valuable, contributing members of the team.

Individual members of the group are encouraged and expected to take risks and try new roles, even though they may fail. For example, a relatively new nurse may be asked to head up an ad hoc committee that is charged to look at how the working relationships between licensed and unlicensed personnel can be enhanced. With the guidance and support of the nurse manager or more seasoned nurses on the unit, this new nurse would be expected to take the lead in working with group members to formulate the goals for this group, suggesting ways the group could go about achieving those goals, maintaining open communications with other nurses not directly involved in the project about the progress of the committee, and keeping the group focused on preparing a timely report that includes realistic, feasible recommendations for how working relationships can be

"I view mistakes as opportunities to learn."

—Zerrie Campbell

enhanced. Along the way, this nurse may make some mistakes, but he or she has been provided with an opportunity to develop leadership skills and to think of himself or herself as a leader.

An environment that facilitates leadership development does not "recycle" the same people over and again, giving only a limited number of individuals an opportunity to grow. Although there is some merit in "recycling" leaders (Kelly, 1991; Stocker, 1991) (e.g., organizations that do this make the best use of people who have proven themselves to be effective, and they benefit from the experience and history of these individuals), repeated recycling with limited opportunities for involvement of inexperienced nurses does not serve the profession well in the long run because it does little to contribute to the ongoing development of leaders.

Finally, a leadership development environment is characterized by good channels of communication and a sense that all members are free to suggest ideas (e.g., they do not merely wait for the person "in charge" to generate ideas). It "forces" members to address issues of significance to them and the profession, and it encourages the sharing of information, rather than the hoarding of it. The Leadership Environment Assessment Survey (Table 9–1) can be used to help analyze the extent to which one's work settings or the professional organizations in which one is involved facilitate the development of leadership.

Empowerment

The environment that encourages, supports, and expects leadership development can be thought of as an empowering environment. Empowerment is a process in which individuals feel strengthened, in control, and in possession of some degree of power. It often is "given" by someone in a position of power or authority (e.g., a nurse manager, the home health agency supervisor), but it also can be "taken" by an individual.

When someone in a position of power empowers others, it is through the sharing of that power. People are empowered by others when they are invited to participate in making decisions that will affect their lives, their work, and their futures. Rather than having "Big Brother" make all the decisions because "he knows best," those people who will have to live with the consequences of decisions are involved in making them. It is clear that this model has relevance for the administrator–staff nurse relationship, but it also has relevance for the nurse-patient relationship, the teacher-student relationship, the parent-child relationship, and any other relationship in which one person typically has more power than others.

Table 9–1 *Leadership Environment Assessment Survey*

Think about your place of employment or a professional organization in which you are involved (e.g., your state nurses' association, your clinical specialty group, your local honor society). With that organization in mind, consider each of the following questions about the nature of the general environment or "culture." YES responses to most questions suggest that the organization supports, encourages, and expects leadership among its members. NO responses to most questions may suggest that the organization's priorities do not include leadership development.

Question	Yes	No
Is this organization open to new ideas and new ways of doing things?	___	___
Do members of the organization feel free to raise questions about	___	___
what is being done?	___	___
how things are being done?	___	___
why things are being done at all?	___	___
why things are done in a particular way?	___	___
Is a questioning attitude accepted, encouraged, and expected in the organization?	___	___
Does the organization put individuals into "boxes"?	___	___
Does the organization push members to strive for excellence?	___	___
Is competition among group members healthy and productive?	___	___
Are the strengths and talents of individual members recognized?	___	___

Table 9–1 *Leadership Environment Assessment Survey—continued*		
Question	**Yes**	**No**
Are the strengths and talents of individual members built upon?	_____	_____
Are group members expected to guide, encourage, and support each other as they continue to grow?	_____	_____
Are leaders allowed to emerge in the organization?	_____	_____
Are followers seen as valuable, contributing members of the group?	_____	_____
Are individual group members encouraged to take risks and try new things?	_____	_____
Are mistakes accepted as part of the learning process for group members?	_____	_____
Are different group members given opportunities to develop as leaders?	_____	_____
Are channels of communication clear and open?	_____	_____
Are group members allowed and encouraged to address issues that are of significance to them and the profession?	_____	_____
Is information shared?	_____	_____
Are accomplishments of group members acknowledged and rewarded?	_____	_____

Nurses are empowered in their organizations when they are held accountable. Rather than being in a position where blame can be placed on someone else or "the system" for less-than-ideal outcomes, empowered nurses know that the quality of care they deliver is their responsibility and that they are accountable for their actions and inactions. By being held accountable, nurses actually have more power in the practice arena.

Nurses are empowered when a shared governance model is in place. In this environment, nurses set their own schedule, formulate their own goals for their unit or agency, set their own standards of excellence, participate actively in peer review, and support one another. The structure is more open and interactive than limiting and hierarchical, and the success or failure of the group is the responsibility of all members, not only the nurse manager or supervisor. Such a model requires that nurses are adequately prepared to assume such responsibility and that there is a mix of skills and experiences in the group to implement the model most effectively.

Although we tend to think of empowerment as something someone in power does for those who are more powerless, that is far from the only means to empowerment. Nurses who find themselves in work or professional environments that are not designed to be empowering can still feel strengthened and "in control" by their own actions.

Empowerment or strength comes from a number of sources. Among the most significant of those sources is knowledge. Nurses empower themselves when they are knowledgeable and expert in their area of practice: when they know the structure, dynamics, and culture of the organizations in which they work; and when they know how to use resources effectively. They also empower themselves when they know themselves: their strengths and limitations, their values and biases, and what motivates them.

Empowerment also comes from having a sense of control over one's life. This may take the form of choosing where one will work; the level of excellence toward which one will strive, regardless, perhaps, of the standards held by others in the setting; and the degree to which one will accept being spoken down to, taken advantage of, or criticized unjustly. To some extent, it is related to self-esteem, self-worth, personal pride, and one's sense of identity.

> *"The secret of joy in work is contained in one word—excellence. To know how to do something well is to enjoy it."*
> —Pearl Buck

Participating actively in one's work setting, professional association, or community also gives one a sense of having control over one's life and is empowering. By serving on committees, for example, nurses are in a better position to influence decisions that are made, and they are able to ensure that nursing's voice is heard; this is empowering. Holding office in a professional association or engaging actively in the debate of issues presented at a convention of that association is empowering because it gives nurses an opportunity to shape the future of the organization and, perhaps, the profession. Meeting with local legislators and community leaders about ways to enhance the resources available to children and the elderly in one's community is empowering because it reinforces one's ability to advocate for and help improve the lives of those who cannot speak for themselves.

Thus, empowerment need not occur only when someone in a position of power or authority decides to "give" some of that power away. Each of us can "take" some power by our own actions. Perhaps we need to return to school for an advanced degree, attend a workshop on assertiveness, volunteer to serve on a committee, run for political office, or review and reaffirm our values related to excellence and quality patient care. Perhaps we also can feel more empowered by entering into a relationship with a mentor.

Mentoring

Mentor was a figure in Greek mythology who served as the wise and faithful guardian and tutor of Telemachus during the 10-year absence of his father, Odysseus, who fought in and struggled to return home from the Trojan War. The words "mentor" and "mentoring," therefore, typically refer to an experienced individual who befriends and guides a less experienced individual.

Although the word "mentor" is often abused today—with anyone who shows the slightest interest in a person or offers the slightest amount of assistance being referred to as a "mentor"—a true mentor invests a great deal of time and effort in the advancement and growth of a protégé. Such a relationship is a conscious, purposefully designed one that typically extends over a number of years.

WHAT IS A MENTOR?

Mentors are close, trusted, experienced counselors or guides. They are accomplished and more experienced individuals, usually, but not always, in the same profession of the neophyte, and they offer neophytes advice, teach them, sponsor them, and guide them through significant points in their careers. As such, they help protégés establish themselves in the profession.

By serving as a mixture of "good parent" and "good friend," mentors provide counsel during times of stress, encouragement during risk-taking endeavors, intellectual challenges, and assistance in the development and enhancement of professional skills. They encourage, cajole, test, teach by example, advise, model, act as a partner, sponsor, and give honest feedback, both positive and negative.

Mentors see some potential in a neophyte, which the neophyte often does not see in herself or himself, and then they do something about that potential. The "something" mentors do is to commit themselves to the neophytes, often for a number of years:

helping them develop a clearer professional identity, fostering their growth in personal and professional power, supporting and facilitating the realization of their dreams, and acting as an energizer and a sounding board.

Mentors also inspire neophytes and challenge them to achieve a level of professionalism they may not have known otherwise. By representing a point of development to which neophytes aspire, mentors invite their protégés into a new world, as peers and colleagues, and open doors for them. They help their protégés "learn the ropes" within a broadened community of colleagues so that they can sense the political climate, spot the behind-the-scenes actions, gain insights into the profession, and expand their networks.

MYTHS ABOUT MENTORS AND MENTORING

Mentoring often is thought of as a panacea for solving the problems of nurses in the healthcare arena or women executives aspiring to climb the corporate ladder. Nurses, however, would be wise to be alert to a number of myths surrounding mentors and mentoring (Sandler, 1993):

- *Myth: The best way to succeed is to have a mentor.* Reality: Mentoring is important and can make a significant difference in the career development of many individuals, but it is not necessarily essential for success or survival.
- *Myth: Mentoring is always beneficial.* Reality: Although there are numerous benefits to a mentoring relationship, there are some limitations as well, such as the difficulty in sustaining the intensity required of both participants over time, the exclusivity of the relationship (e.g., the mentor invests in a very small number of individuals and is not available to work with a larger number of neophytes), the potential for the protégé to rely primarily or exclusively on the mentor for emotional support and guidance rather than interacting with a broader scope of colleagues, and the fact that the mentor, not the protégé, typically "sets the agenda."
- *Myth: The mentor should be older than the person being mentored.* Reality: It is quite possible that the more experienced, accomplished individual in the relationship is younger chronologically.
- *Myth: A person can have only one mentor at a time.* Reality: Although it may be difficult to maintain close, intense relationships with several mentors simultaneously, it is not impossible. One mentor may be most effective in helping a neophyte write grants, another may be the expert clinician

who gives guidance with difficult clinical problems, and a third may be the best resource in gaining entry to a professional association.

- *Myth: If you are seeking a mentor, you have to wait to be asked.* Reality: It is perfectly acceptable for a neophyte to approach a potential mentor to discuss the possibility of entering into a relationship.
- *Myth: Men are better mentors for women.* Reality: Most mentors throughout history probably have been men largely because women were not socialized (until recently) in the direction of such relationships and there were not many women in positions of leadership to serve as mentors. However, there is no evidence to support the claim that men are better mentors. In fact, with women's tendency to attend to personal issues and not merely work or professional ones, a female mentor may be more effective than a male mentor.
- *Myth: When a man mentors a woman, the chances are great that it will develop into a sexual encounter.* Reality: This, of course, is a possibility in any relationship, but when the mentoring relationship is kept focused on the career development and advancement of the protégé, sexuality need not and, indeed, should not enter into it.
- *Myth: The mentor always knows best.* Reality: Although it is true that the mentor is the wiser, more experienced member of the pair, it also is important to remember that the protégé is a bright, talented individual with ideas and a great deal of potential. Those talents should not be ignored or exploited in the relationship to benefit or stroke the ego of the mentor. The whole point of a mentoring relationship is to promote the career advancement of the protégé, not to make the protégé dependent on the mentor. Thus the protégé must play a significant role in the relationship and sometimes is the person who "knows best."

WHAT MENTORS LOOK FOR IN PROTÉGÉS

Mentors and leaders look for novices who have the potential to move the profession ahead. They then invest the time, energy, and caring to create what they believe will be a future leader in the field. With this kind of investment expected of mentors, it is no wonder that they would choose neophytes who show they are worth investing in and are likely to show some measure of "return on the investment."

Specifically, mentors often seek protégés who possess certain qualities. Table 9–2 presents characteristics that may serve as a

Table 9–2 *What Mentors Look for in Protégés*

Mentors often seek protégés who possess certain qualities. The following characteristics may serve as a guide to determine whether you are the kind of individual in whom a mentor might invest:

- Intelligence
- A self-starter: someone who is internally motivated
- Someone who is looking for new challenges
- Good interpersonal and communication skills: someone who is articulate
- A risk-taker
- A hard worker
- Someone who has and understands ideas and is always open to new ideas and possibilities
- Integrity
- Someone who presents himself or herself professionally: in appearance, through the written word, and so on
- A sense of humor
- Someone who is willing to invest in himself or herself
- A curious mind: someone who asks questions and is not satisfied with the status quo
- Someone who has a vision: for himself or herself and for the profession

guide for each of us to determine whether we are the kind of individual in whom a mentor might invest. In essence, mentors look for protégés who are beginning leaders or have the potential to be leaders. They then work to help those individuals develop the knowledge, skills, and savvy needed to be effective leaders.

CAVEATS REGARDING A MENTOR RELATIONSHIP

When considering entering a mentoring relationship, both individuals should consider the following caveats or "commandments" (Sandler, 1993):

- Be careful not to confuse a mentor relationship with a personal, emotional one.

- Many people can be mentors—you need not be at the top of your profession to be of assistance to novices.
- The protégé must take personal responsibility for learning.
- The mentor should not be expected to fulfill every need and meet every demand of the protégé.
- The confidences of the mentor must be respected.
- Expectations of both the mentor and protégé (e.g., time, type of assistance) need to be clarified early on in the relationship.
- Protégés should know if they are asking for too much, or too little, of the mentor.
- The feedback from the mentor to the protégé should take the form of praise and constructive criticism, with specific suggestions for improvement.
- The relationship should be used to open doors for future protégés.
- Mentors and protégés need not come from the same type of educational, ethnic, racial, religious, or any other type of background.
- Recognize that the relationship goes through stages— from dependence, uncertainty, and hesitancy to mutual give-and-take to termination, at which point the protégé is more independent and identifies his or her separateness from the mentor.
- Be careful not to fall into mentoring because "it's the thing to do" or the "in" thing.

BENEFITS TO THE MENTOR

Although it may sound as if the only person who benefits from a mentor relationship is the protégé, nothing could be further from the truth. Indeed, mentoring is a mutually supportive, mutually beneficial relationship in which the mentor also gains a great deal.

The strength of mentors comes from their own professional experience, self-worth, and autonomy. They must be capable of motivating neophytes to be creative and possess a good sense of their own creative selves. But they also must be careful not to direct or control every facet of their protégé's life, and they must be open and willing to learn from the protégé.

As the individuals engage in this evolving relationship, the protégé often pursues more sophisticated lines of investigation, develops skills the mentor may not possess, and establishes new networks. The mentor who is open to and willing to learn from a protégé will grow enormously from the relationship.

It is incredibly rewarding for mentors to see novice prac-titioners, educators, researchers, administrators, and leaders grow and evolve. In many cases, the accomplishments of the neophytes far surpass those of the mentors, and mentors take great pride in seeing their protégés receive awards, make changes in practice, receive offers of significant positions, be elected to office in professional associations, receive competitive grants, and publish articles or books that influence others.

Thus mentors benefit greatly from working with protégés. The true mentoring relationship is mutually rewarding and results in growth in both individuals. In addition to the personal growth one experiences, both individuals also expand their networks of professional colleagues and "influentials."

Networking

As noted, a mentoring relationship can help both participants develop contacts and expand their professional networks, networks they may call on throughout their careers for assistance, support of ideas, and guidance. Although some take offense at the idea of "using" people to one's benefit, the whole concept of networking is built on the assumption that who one knows is important and can be helpful.

Networks form for the purpose of providing access to contacts, referrals, information, support, feedback, understanding, and empathy. They also can serve to help nurses maintain a social and professional identity and provide a means of working toward organizational, professional, or societal reform.

Nurses might "tap into" their networks when they are looking for a guest speaker for a program, a consultant, someone to fill a key position in an organization, someone to nominate for appointment to a community board, or an expert in a clinical area. They might also use their networks to gather data about practices in other institutions that can help advance a proposal for a change in their own institutions. Thus networks serve a number of useful purposes, without the sustained, intense investment of a mentor relationship.

As described, mentoring is a special kind of relationship between two individuals that is intense, personalized, and long-lasting and that has positive outcomes for both participants. Indeed, studies have documented several positive outcomes from engagement in a mentoring relationship.

In a classic study of 1250 top executives, Roche (1979) found that almost two-thirds of those studied had mentors, and most mentoring relationships started when the protégé was in his or her twenties or thirties. Roche found that executives who had mentors moved into successful positions more quickly, earned more money at a younger age, were more likely to follow a personal career plan, were better educated, were more satisfied with their career progress, received greater pleasure from their work, and eventually sponsored protégés themselves.

In a classic study of 71 nurse influentials, Vance (1977) found that 83 percent of those studied had mentors, and 93 percent of them were consciously aware of being mentors to others. A follow-up study (Kinsey, 1986) revealed similar findings, namely, that many of those nurses who were thought of as influentials in the profession had, themselves, been mentored by others and had served as mentors to novices.

But does everyone need a mentor to "make it" and "get ahead"? The answer, without question, is "No." However, most people do need guides, support systems, sounding boards, and peer "pals" to help during certain times throughout their careers, and this is where one's network can be most effective.

Peer "pals" are peers who help each other. For example, nurses may help each other manage a particularly difficult community health problem or deal with an arrogant physician. Guides are people who know easier ways to do something or have experienced a particular situation and share those insights with others. For example, nurses who are enrolled in a master's program may serve as guides to colleagues who are in the process of deciding whether they should pursue graduate education and, if so, what school to attend and what specialty to pursue; or nurses who have particularly good writing skills may review and critique an abstract before it is submitted in response to a "call" for presentation at a conference or a manuscript before it is submitted to a journal for review. Sponsors are individuals who will act on behalf of others, promote them, and advance them, much the same way a mentor does, but in more isolated instances, rather than over a lengthy period. For example, a faculty member may nominate a graduate for an award or suggest that graduate as a candidate for office in a professional association. All of these are examples of a patron-type system in which nurses "use" their networks but do not necessarily enter into an extended, intense mentoring relationship.

CONCLUSION

The development of leadership knowledge and skills throughout one's career requires (1) purposeful, goal-directed action; (2) honest, extensive self-assessment; (3) a willingness to ask for assistance or guidance; and (4) a willingness to accept help or guidance when it is offered. It is enhanced by the development and effective use of professional networks, as well as engagement in mentoring relationships.

Nurses who are in positions of influence must take on the responsibility of grooming other promising nurses. Those seeking to be more influential and become leaders must start early to seek experiences and colleagues—and possibly mentors—who will provide the professional and personal nourishment necessary for success. We must identify the people we know who are in a position to help us, let them know we respect their ability, and seek their support. We also must help them see that they have something to gain by helping and guiding and possibly mentoring us.

> *"Whatever development process you're comfortable with, do it to the maximum."*
>
> —Bonnie Saucier

Each of us must create a personal plan for leadership development throughout our careers and then take responsibility for implementing that plan. Such a plan may include advancing our formal education or enrolling in courses or workshops that will help us develop a better understanding of the phenomenon of leadership or specific skills, such as assertiveness or public speaking. It may include looking for a work setting or professional association that is empowering or one in which strong role models exist. Our personal plan for leadership development may incorporate seeking a mentor, expanding our professional networks, becoming more involved in the political process, running for office in our specialty organization, submitting a manuscript for publication, or responding to a call for paper presentations at a regional or national conference.

Whatever the specific course of action, we will develop as leaders through a well-thought-out plan, and not through the waving of some magic wand. Taking responsibility is a large part of what leadership is all about. And taking responsibility for our own development as leaders is an excellent way to achieve our professional goals more effectively.

Critical Thinking 9–1

Critical Thinking Exercises

Read at least three journal editorials, one by Leah Curtin, one by Barbara Stevens Barnum, and one by another editor. To what extent do these individuals express controversial ideas and convey a passion about their topic? Do you see any difference in the uniqueness of perspective, challenging nature of the ideas put forth, or passion expressed by the editors? What can you learn from this comparison about the nature of risk taking that is inherent in a leadership role? If you were given the opportunity to write a controversial editorial for a prominent nursing journal, what would you write about? How would you express your ideas? Who would you ask to review your manuscript before you submitted it?

_____

_____

Complete the Leadership Environment Assessment Survey. To what extent does "your" organization provide an environment that promotes leadership? What can you do to make "your" environment more conducive to the development of leadership skills?

_____

_____

Review the discussion about "what mentors look for in a protégé." How do you "rate" in each of the areas listed? What assets do you think you would bring to a mentoring relationship?

_____

_____

List the qualities you would like to see in your mentor. Who do you know—in your immediate environment, from your educational program, in your specialty organization, in your local community, through your professional readings—that possesses all or most of those qualities? Consider making a contact with that person to discuss the possibility of establishing a mentoring relationship.

_____

_____

The next time you attend a professional conference or convention, make it a point to meet at least three new colleagues. Talk to each one about his or her interests, areas of expertise, goals, current position, and so on. You also should be prepared to discuss these same points. Exchange e-mail addresses or obtain a business card from each new colleague; note pertinent information about the individual, along with the date and conference where you met the individual; and file it when you return home. This will help you build your professional network.

_____

_____

Write your personal career goals: What position would you like to hold 25 years from now? What types of offices would you like to hold? What awards would you like to have won or honors to have been bestowed on you? What types of books or articles would you like to have published? What would you like to be "known for" in the nursing community? How influential would you like to be on the local, national, and international level? Think big! Now, for each goal, list the types of actions you will need to take to achieve that goal, and plot a timeline for each action. For example, if you would like to publish an article in _Image: The Journal of Nursing Scholarship_, you may want to take an intensive writing course; read carefully the articles published in that journal in the last 5 years to better understand the nature of what is published and its format; take a paper you wrote for school or a difficult, challenging patient case study you presented at rounds and rewrite to fit the guidelines of that journal; submit that paper to a former faculty member or a trusted colleague at work for critique and comment; talk to other nurses who have published in _Image_ or other prestigious journals about their experience "breaking into" the publication arena; seek a mentor to assist you with writing for publication; and so on.

_____

_____

References

Annual Report 1998. (1999). Indianapolis: Sigma Theta Tau International.

Ferguson, S.L. (1998). Academy, Foundation launch program to enhance nurses' leadership capacity. *The American Nurse 30*(4), 10.

Kelly, L.S. (1991). The conundrum of recycled leadership (Editorial). *Nursing Outlook 39*(1), 5.

Kelley, R. (1992). *The power of followership: How to create leaders people want to follow and followers who lead themselves.* New York: Doubleday Currency.

Kinsey, D.C. (1986). The new nurse influentials. *Nursing Outlook 34*(5), 238–240.

Reisberg, L. (1998). Students gain sense of direction in new field of leadership studies. *Chronicle of Higher Education 45*(10), A49–A50.

Roche, G. (1979). Much ado about mentors. *Harvard Business Review 58,* 14ff.

Sandler, B.R. (1993). Women as mentors: Myths and commandments (Opinion). *The Chronicle of Higher Education 39*(27), B3.

Schwartz, M.K. (Ed.). (1998). *Leadership education: A source book of courses and programs.* Greensboro, NC: Center for Creative Leadership.

Stocker, S. (1991). Unraveling the leadership conundrum (Sounding Board). *Nursing Outlook 39*(4), 188–189.

Vance, C.N. (1977). *A group profile of contemporary influentials in American nursing.* Unpublished doctoral dissertation, Teachers College, Columbia University, New York.

Bibliography

Bos, S. (1998). Perceived benefits of peer leadership as described by junior baccalaureate nursing students. *Journal of Nursing Education 37*(4), 189–191.

Curtin, L. (1993). Empowerment: On eagles' wings (Editorial). *Nursing Management 24*(6), 7–8.

Fields, W.L. (1991). Mentoring in nursing: A historical approach. *Nursing Outlook 39,* 257–281.

Gibson, C.H. (1991). A concept analysis of empowerment. *Journal of Advanced Nursing 16,* 354–361.

Glennon, T.K. (1992). Empowering nurses through enlightened leadership. *The Journal of Nurse Empowerment 2*(1), 41–44.

Gunden, E., & Crissman, S. (1992). Leadership skills for empowerment. *Nursing Administration Quarterly 16*(3), 6–10.

Hartshorn, J.C., Berbiglia, V.A., & Heye, M. (1997). An honors program: Directing our future leaders. *Journal of Nursing Education 36*(4), 187–189.

Helmuth, M. (1994). Mock convention: A simulation for teaching leadership. *Journal of Nursing Education 33*(4), 159–160.

Kessenich, C.R. (1997). The evolution of a leadership course. *Journal of Nursing Education 36*(6), 301–303.

Krichbaum, K. (1997). Preparing students for leadership in practice. *Creative Nursing 2,* 12–14.

McCall, M.W., Jr. (1998). *High flyers: Developing the next generation of leaders.* Boston: Harvard Business School Press.

Olson, R.K., & Vance, C.N. (1993). *Mentorship in nursing: A collection of research abstracts with selected bibliographies—1977–1992.* Houston: University of Texas Printing Services.

Prestholdt, C.O. (1990). Modern mentoring: Strategies for developing contemporary nursing leadership. *Nursing Administration Quarterly 15*(1), 20–27.

Stewart, B.M., & Krueger, L.E. (1996). An evolutionary concept analysis of mentoring in nursing. *Journal of Professional Nursing 12*(5), 311–321.

Taylor, D.E., Barrick, C.B., & Harrell, F.H. (1994). Preparing students for health care reform: An innovative approach for teaching leadership/management. *Journal of Nursing Education 33*(5), 230–232.

Tebbitt, B.V. (1993). Demystifying organizational empowerment. *Journal of Nursing Administration 23*(1), 18–23.

Vance, C., & Olson, R.K. (Eds.). (1998). *The mentor connection in nursing.* New York: Springer.

Wilson, B., & Laschinger, H.K. (1994). Staff nurse perception of job empowerment and organizational commitment. *Journal of Nursing Administration 24*(4), 39–47.

Yoder, L. (1990). Mentoring: A concept analysis. *Nursing Administration Quarterly 15*(1), 9–19.

CHAPTER 10

Conclusions

The New Leadership Challenge, Excellence, and Professional Involvement

Conclusions

The New Leadership Challenge, Excellence, and Professional Involvement

Learning Objectives

☐ Analyze the concept of excellence.

☐ Discuss the responsibility leaders who will create nursing's preferred future have for promoting excellence.

☐ Examine the interrelationship among leadership, excellence, and professional involvement.

☐ Propose strategies for exercising leadership, promoting excellence, and being professionally involved to create nursing's preferred future.

INTRODUCTION

One of the responsibilities of those leaders who will create nursing's preferred future is to promote excellence. As nursing professionals, we certainly have a responsibility to strive for excellence in our own practice and in the delivery of healthcare to consumers. But as leaders who will create a future for nursing that acknowledges and takes full advantage of the myriad talents nurses bring to the healthcare arena, we have an even greater responsibility to promote excellence.

This chapter examines the concept of excellence in depth. Excellence is then related to leadership, and the role of leaders in advancing the notion of excellence is explored. Finally, both concepts— excellence and leadership—are blended with the idea of professional involvement throughout one's career as a means to promote nursing and create a preferred future for our profession.

> *"The rewards of excellence do not come easily; it requires rigorous discipline to achieve them."*
> —Edgar Dale

The Concept of Excellence

"Excellence" is a word we hear tossed about everywhere recently. General Motors says they are in the business of excellence. IBM claims they are all about excellence. The American Nurses Association (ANA) talks about excellence in clinical practice. The National League for Nursing (NLN) promotes excellence in nursing education. Sigma Theta Tau International advances excellence in scholarship. And our colleges and universities talk about excellence in their program offerings, faculty, students, and facilities. But what is excellence? What is meant by this often-used but little-examined word?

Excellence means striving to be the very best you can be in everything you do—not because some teacher or parent or other "authority" figure pushes you to do that, but because you cannot imagine functioning in any other way. It means setting high standards for yourself and the groups in which you are involved, holding yourself to those standards despite challenges or pressures to reduce or lower them, and not being satisfied with anything less than the very best.

This kind of perspective or approach applies to all spheres of life—writing papers for a course, preparing for a final examination, providing care to elderly patients in a long-term care facility, teaching school-age children about good nutrition or sexually transmitted diseases, driving a car, or working to secure more resources for the

"In all that you do, reflect the excellence that's in you."
—Martin Luther King

homeless in our community. Individuals who are committed to excellence do not—and will not—settle for second best, mediocre performance, or "getting by."

When we allow ourselves and the systems in which we function to simply be "OK," "good enough," or minimally adequate, we sell ourselves short, and we do little to advance the profession of nursing and ensure quality of care for patients, families, and communities. We fail to be challenged, we fail to grow, we fail to make change, and we fail to help others develop. Excellence means not allowing this state of affairs to exist!

Excellence also means being unwilling to accept the status quo. This does not mean that all one does is criticize the way things are being done and then walk away in the hopes that someone else will correct what is wrong. Instead, individuals who strive for and expect excellence question and challenge the status quo by asking why things are done the way they are, examining the assumptions that underlie existing practices, and offering thoughtful and realistic alternatives for how things could be done in other ways. They then also are willing to invest the time and energy to implement those alternatives, evaluate their effectiveness, and orchestrate change so that those new approaches become integral to the system.

Excellence means to excel—to surpass—to be the best. It can be equated with accuracy, flawlessness, and even perfection—terms with which many of us are uncomfortable. Indeed, for many, perfection and the pursuit of excellence represents the "impossible dream." But in an article about perfection in organizations, Mescon and Mescon (1984) noted that "the pursuit of perfection is a challenge and a chase that must be won. . . . We must put to rest the notion that excellence represents fantasy, not fact in organizational life

"Look for the ideal, but put it into the actual."
—Florence Nightingale

today" (p. 94). Perhaps this statement could be modified to say that "we must put to rest the notion that excellence represents fantasy, not fact in [nursing practice] today!" According to these authors, "nothing but perfection is acceptable, [and] nothing but perfection should be rewarded" (p. 94).

> *"Let me tell you the secret that has led me to my goal. My strength lies solely in my tenacity."*
> —Louis Pasteur

Excellence is not an "impossible dream." In fact, if we look at just what excellence is, we see it is not so foreign or so unattainable. Many people have written about excellence, but the description of that concept offered by Diers and Evans (1980) is particularly helpful. These authors say that excellence involves several things:

- *Discipline:* drawing on our knowledge and experience to practice in a "systematic" way that is of the highest caliber; in other words, "not settling for second best"
- *Choreography:* successfully balancing competing demands in our pursuit of goals
- *Responsibility:* acknowledging what we have done well or poorly and blaming no one
- *Caring—consistently:* demonstrating a concern and a compassion for others (including our colleagues) and for ourselves
- *Skepticism:* keeping a proper distance from the truth and not accepting everything blindly; keeping our minds open to new ideas, new information, and new approaches
- *Perseverance:* continually striving to fulfill a goal or realize a vision
- *Passion:* "the essence of excellence"; being "inflamed" by our work

Diers and Evans (1980) say "excellent nurses are inflamed by nursing . . . To be an excellent nurse is to be suffused with a deep and almost inexpressible passion for humankind" (p. 30).

Quality is never an accident. It is always the result of high intention, sincere effort, intelligent direction, and skillful execution. It represents the wise choice of many alternatives.

A commitment to pursuing excellence does not just happen; it does not just randomly occur. Doing whatever it is that must

> *"Excellence is the gradual result of always striving to do better."*
> —Pat Riley

be done requires an ongoing attention that is initiated and maintained by top management in an organization. Management also recruits and may even reward individuals who are committed to excellence and who consistently produce excellent work. But achieving excellence occurs only with individual investment. Top management and "the organization" can do only so much. What each of us needs to remember is that every job is a self-portrait of the person who did it. Each of us needs to autograph our work with excellence.

The pursuit of excellence must be vigorously and relentlessly incorporated into everything we think, say, and do. As Mescon and Mescon (1984) wrote, "it is the little things that count on the road to perfection. But too often it is the little things that we all too often simply forget" (p. 94). The individual who autographs his or her work with excellence does not ignore or forget the little things, just as he or she does not forget the big ones.

Vince Lombardi, former coach of the Green Bay Packers football team, once said, "The quality of a person's life is in direct proportion to his or her commitment to excellence, regardless of the chosen field of endeavor." This is a profound concept when one considers the significant role it suggests excellence plays in our lives.

According to Gardner (1961), "We must learn to honor excellence (indeed to demand it) in every socially accepted human activity, however humble the activity, and to scorn shoddiness, however exalted the activity. An excellent plumber is infinitely more admirable than an incompetent philosopher. The society which scorns excellence in plumbing because plumbing is a humble activity and tolerates shoddiness in philosophy because it is an exalted activity will have neither good plumbing nor good philosophy. Neither its pipes nor its theories will hold water" (p. 102).

> "If a man is called to be a streetsweeper, he should sweep streets even as Michelangelo painted or Beethoven composed music, or Shakespeare wrote poetry. He should sweep streets so well that all the hosts of heaven and earth will pause to say, here lived a great streetsweeper who did his job well."
>
> —Martin Luther King

Each of us who hopes to make a significant contribution to our organization, our profession, our community, or the world needs to make this commitment. The quality of our lives will be enhanced as a result. As Aristotle said, we are what we repeatedly do. Excellence, then, is not an isolated act, but a habit.

As mentioned earlier, excellence needs to be a way of life, and for those who do make it a habit, it sets up a "vicious cycle." In other words, excellence begets excellence—for ourselves and for those around us.

This striving for excellence is highly contagious because peer pressure and collegial influence have powerful effects and because they can usually do more than management ever could. Evidence exists to support this claim. Curtain (1990) reported on studies that showed that nurses who practice on units where excellent nursing is the norm soon are striving and growing to reach the level of excellence demonstrated by their peers. However, when nurses practice on a unit where the standard of care is poor and everyone is satisfied merely with maintaining the status quo and "getting by," their practice tends to descend to the lowest common denominator on that unit. Thus the level of excellence found in practice is a function of the collegiality among nurses and the kind of "habits" they have. It is a reflection of the way they challenge and support each other, and the way they practice, repeatedly.

> *"I never had a policy: I have just tried to do my best each and every day."*
> —Abraham Lincoln

Perhaps each of us needs to take what has been referred to as "the mirror test." Look at ourselves in a mirror and ask if we can honestly tell the person we see there that we have done our very best.

Excellence comes from within, and perfection is impossible without that personal investment. If staff tolerate mediocrity in what they do, practice will be mediocre. Management can create an environment that expects, fosters, and rewards excellence, but it is only when each individual in the organization can "pass the mirror test" and honestly say that he or she has done his or her very best that excellence will occur.

Unless we try to do something beyond what we have already mastered, we will never grow. Excellence involves challenging ourselves—accepting challenges that are offered to us (e.g., writing a grant proposal, pursuing advancement through the agency's clinical levels, facilitating a research project on your unit, accepting an invitation to speak at a professional meeting or to the media). Excellence also involves seeking new experiences (e.g., asking to serve on a committee, agreeing to have one's name placed on a ballot for election to a committee or office, assuming new responsibilities with cross-training, submitting an abstract in response to a call for papers). Excellence is not allowing ourselves to get too comfortable or too complacent or so wrapped up in our "little corner of the world" that we lose that broader perspective.

No one ever attains very eminent success by simply doing what is required of her or him. It is the amount and excellence of what is done over and above the required that determines the greatness of ultimate distinction.

In our society and in nursing, we have, for too long, accepted the mundane, promoted the average, and rewarded the mediocre. But the organization or the profession that is going to make a difference—to the recipients of its services and to those providing the service—is the one that prizes the absolute best at all levels. It is the organization that never forgets the ideal of excellence and never loses the aspiration to go beyond the merely "acceptable."

It has been said that only those who dare to fail greatly can ever achieve greatly. In other words, it is only when we strive for excellence, for flawlessness, and for perfection that we will achieve it. In that process we may fail; therefore, taking risks is a critical component of achieving excellence. Yes, we may fail along the way, but we need to try because excellence also involves action. One anonymous writer put this idea into words by saying that "Some people dream of worthy accomplishments while others stay awake and actually do them."

Having a dream is critical, but it is not enough. Each of us needs to be able to articulate that dream clearly, express it to others, and entice others to work with us to make it become reality. This is the essence of leadership.

Leadership and Excellence

Just as excellence is a complex phenomenon, so too is leadership. As noted earlier, Burns (1978, p. 2), asserted that "leadership is one of the most observed and least understood phenomena on earth." Despite this lack of full understanding, however, many elements of leadership are universal, elements that bear reviewing.

First, there is agreement that, unlike management, *leadership is not necessarily tied to a position of authority in an organization.* One can be a leader as a staff nurse or as a student, just as well as if one is a nurse manager, the vice president for nursing, a faculty member, a

> *"The secret to leadership is ... bearing the larger picture always in mind. Ask yourself, 'What are we really trying to accomplish?'"*
> —J. Donald Walters

dean, or the president of a professional association. In fact, it may be easier to be a leader if one is not in a position of authority because then that individual is not expected to promote any "party line," and it may be easier for him or her to "rock the boat" by raising difficult questions, articulating a vision, and working toward changing the system.

Second, *leadership is a relationship of influence,* more than a relationship of authority. People follow leaders by choice, not because they are required to do so.

Perhaps one of the most important characteristics of leaders is that *leaders have a vision;* they see new possibilities, new horizons, and different options. They have some notion of things being able to be better than they are now, regardless of how good they are now. In addition, this vision is their cause or purpose in life, and they are willing to invest enormous amounts of energy to see it re-alized. Think again about Martin Luther King, Jr., who worked all his life for racial equality and the peaceful resolution of differences. Or think about Mother Teresa, who devoted her life to helping the poor and disenfranchised; or Candy Lightner, who lost her daughter to a drunk driver and ended up establishing Mothers Against Drunk Driving (MADD); or any number of other individuals who had a vision of a better world and worked to see it materialize. This is the stuff of which leaders are made. Each of us needs to ask if we are leaders—if we have a vision of a better world.

> *"In the quiet hours when we are alone and there is nobody to tell us what fine fellows we are, we come sometimes upon a moment in which we wonder, not how much money we are earning, nor how famous we have become, but what good we are doing."*
>
> —A.A. Milne

In accord with this drive toward realizing a vision, *leaders are change agents.* They are innovators who continually challenge the status quo, who are willing to stick their heads above the crowd and take the risk of being shot down. They strive to keep people and organizations moving forward. Again, each of us needs to ask ourselves if we are leaders—if we work toward positive change.

If leaders are going to be agents of change, they also must be *comfortable with conflict.* In fact, leaders must be able and willing to seek conflict, introduce it if necessary, and use it to achieve the goals of the group. They do not always want to minimize conflict or "sweep it under the rug" because they know that conflict is healthy and it promotes growth in individuals and organizations. Ask yourself if you are a leader—if you can manage the conflict we face in our daily lives and our professional lives.

Leaders are *willing to use intuition* in making decisions, they are *comfortable with ambiguity and uncertainty,* and they are *creative.* They want to see new forms take shape, and they do not need to rely on predictability or rationality. They *see the "big picture,"* are *"telescopic,"* seem to *have a "get-it-all-together" perspective,* and *want to collaborate* with others to achieve goals, rather than having a narrow, limited, self-centered interest or focus. Each of us needs to ask ourselves if we are leaders, if we are creative, if we can tolerate uncertainty, and if we can look beyond our own needs.

Finally, leaders are *characterized by excellence,* and they work to promote excellence in themselves and others. Driven by their vision, they strive to be the best they can be, and they inspire others to do the same. Dissatisfied with the status quo, they take risks, try innovative approaches, call on their creativity, and work to make change. Energized by a desire to continue to grow and learn, they seek new opportunities, take on challenges, and know how to manage conflict. Appreciative of the diverse and complex world in which we live, they do not allow themselves to become too highly specialized or too narrowly focused.

Leaders promote and create excellence. And leaders create the future.

Ilona Herlinger (1990, p. 4), former president of the interdisciplinary honor society of Phi Kappa Phi, challenged members of that organization to think about what role they would play during the twenty-first century. The questions she posed are challenges leaders must accept:

- Will you make a significant contribution to or an important difference in the world?
- Will you be a doer or merely an observer?
- Will you be an actor or merely a member of the audience?

In essence, Herlinger challenges us to ponder whether we will strive for excellence or accept mediocrity. She also suggests that we need to consider whether we will be leaders or apathetic, passive crowd-followers.

Professional Involvement

When one thinks about the history of Sigma Theta Tau International, the Honor Society of Nursing, and about the interdisciplinary Honor Society of Phi Kappa Phi, one is inspired by what could be characterized as true leadership and true excellence. Sigma Theta Tau was started in 1922 by six students who wanted to create some way to recognize and acknowledge nursing scholarship. Phi Kappa Phi was started in 1897 by one young man who dreamed of scholars from all disciplines being recognized on college campuses to the same extent that athletes were recognized. Those six students and that one young man each had a vision, they banded together or enlisted the support of others, they took action and worked tirelessly, and they formed two of the most prestigious honor societies in our country.

Today, each of these organizations has hundreds of chapters and thousands of members. They are dedicated to scholarship and leadership (in the case of Sigma Theta Tau) and to promoting academic excellence (in the case of Phi Kappa Phi). They are proactive and forward-looking. Sigma Theta Tau is international in scope and purpose. Each organization is clear about its purpose, each is focused in its efforts, and each is highly regarded, well-respected, and emulated. All of this from a handful of students who saw a need, had a vision, believed in excellence, and exercised leadership.

Members of Sigma Theta Tau are among the most powerful "movers and shakers" in our field. Dorothy Brooten's research on the effects of nursing care on low-birth-weight infants who have been discharged early from the neonatal intensive care unit to home has received accolades from the nursing and medical professions. Lois Evans and Neville Strumpf's extensive work on restraint-free care of the elderly has humanized that care in countless ways. Imogene King's contributions in theory development have been significant in advancing the science of nursing. Melanie Dreher's commitment to advancing the concept of clinical scholarship has been influential in helping nurses in practice develop more significant insights to their practice and be creative in where and how they deliver quality care. And the late Virginia Henderson helped us crystallize the professional nursing role in a way few others have.

> *"Real leaders are ordinary people with extraordinary determination."*
> —Anonymous

By being involved in organizations like this—or in many other professional organizations—each of us has the opportunity to interact with and learn from outstanding individuals. We have the opportunity to see true leaders "in action," connect with and seek possible mentors, be involved in activities that promote excellence, and learn more about ourselves as potential leaders. Individuals such as these have an intense passion for the profession and their own area of work, and they do not hesitate to reach out to, guide, and help others in the field. They share a commitment to advancing the profession in whatever way they can, and they want to invest in others.

Professional involvement also means participating in organizational, community, and political activities to advance our vision and see it become a reality. Nurses who serve on committees where they work, on the board of the local community health center, on school boards, as local freeholders or mayors, or as United States senators, all are in positions of influence and have many opportunities to promote excellence, exercise leadership, and create a preferred future for nursing.

> *"Complexity and collaboration are two sides of the same coin."*
> —Kathleen Dracup (Nurse)

Nurses who publish or give presentations in which controversial ideas are presented or where a high standard of practice is put forth are helping create nursing's preferred future. The same is true for nurses who conduct special projects (funded or not), conduct research and disseminate the findings, mentor others, and engage in collaborative practice with other nurses and with members of other healthcare disciplines. The opportunities to promote excellence and function as a leader are limitless, and each time a nurse engages in activities that advance nursing or that demonstrate leadership to realize a vision, he or she is contributing to the creation of a preferred future for our profession.

CONCLUSION

As we develop as leaders, each of us should take advantage of the opportunities presented to become involved professionally. We might even create opportunities to become involved. Each of us has a responsibility to participate and to try to make a difference. Through networking, role modeling, mentoring relationships, and the continued study of leadership and excellence, practice will be enhanced and we will grow enormously. The outcome will be excellence in our spheres of practice and a preferred future for the nursing profession that we helped create.

> *"When we do the best we can, we never know what miracle is wrought in our life, or in the life of another."*
> —Helen Keller

In conclusion, a contemporary piece of advice seems to capture the essence of leadership, excellence, and professional involvement:

Excellence can be attained if you . . .

> CARE more than others think is wise,
> RISK more than others think is safe,
> DREAM more than others think is practical, and
> EXPECT more than others think is possible.

We hope each student and staff nurse who reads this book will take on the challenges of excellence and leadership. You are the future of our marvelous profession. We have every confidence that you will take up this challenge with all seriousness and that you will succeed in creating a preferred future for nursing.

Critical Thinking Exercises

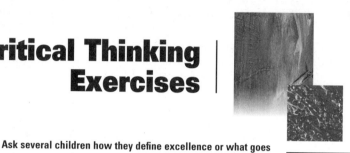

Ask several children how they define excellence or what goes into something being called "excellent." Pose this same question to nurses in practice and to individuals engaged in other professional roles (e.g., teacher, physician, social worker). What common themes emerge in the responses you receive? Are there any differences in the way various groups (e.g., children versus adults, women versus men, nurses versus other professionals) talk about the concept? What conclusions can you draw about why the commonalities and differences exist?

Read a short story or poem or watch a film that has recently received a significant award for excellence, and do the same for a "nonwinner" in the genre. What sets the "winner" apart from the "nonwinner"? What were or seem to be the criteria used to determine excellence in the area? How do those criteria compare to your personal description/definition of excellence?

Identify a nurse who recently received an award that acknowledges excellence—in clinical practice, in education, in research, in contributions to the profession, in the care of a particular population (e.g., the homeless), and so on. The award can be local, regional, national, or international. Interview the award recipient about his or her recognition. Talk about the individual's background, philosophy, accomplishments, contributions, and ideas about excellence and leadership. What have you learned from this interview that you can use to promote excellence and exert leadership in your arena of practice? Outline specific strategies that could lead you to receive such an award in the future.

References

Burns, J.M. (1978). *Leadership.* New York: Harper Torchbooks.

Curtain, L. (1990). The excellence within (Editorial Opinion). *Nursing Management, 21,* 7.

Diers, D., & Evans, D.L. (1980). Excellence in nursing (Editorial). *Image, 12*(2), 27–30.

Gardner, J. (1961). *Excellence.* New York: Harper & Row.

Herlinger, I. (1990). President's corner. *Phi Kappa Phi Newsletter 16,* 4.

Mescon, M.H., & Mescon, T.S. (1984). Perfection: The possible dream. *Sky* (Delta Airlines magazine), *13*(9), 94, 96.

Glossary

Advocate: helping others grow; facilitating growth in others; speaking or acting on behalf of others who cannot speak or act for themselves

Androgyny: blending of assertiveness, competitiveness, and dominance with regard for relationships and cooperativeness

Autocratic/authoritarian leadership style: a dictator-like style that does not involve any participation from the group

Behavioral objective: learner's goal, including desired behavior, evaluation method proposed to measure whether the behavior has been accomplished or not, and target date or time for completion of behavior

Change process: the deliberate application of an intervention(s) to produce an alternative method

Chaos Theory: belief that hidden within the seemingly total disorganization of a situation are patterns of order

Cognitive development: a series of stages through which one progresses from seeing knowledge as finite to viewing knowledge as relative

Collaboration: representatives of several disciplines coming together to jointly solve problems and assist a patient in attaining improved outcomes

Collective bargaining: the process by which employers and employees communicate through union representatives

Conflict management: the negotiation of a potentially win/win, win/lose, or lose/lose situation between two individuals or two groups

Credibility: competency, honest, vision, and inspiration

Cross-trained: a process by which staff are inserviced to work competently on two different patient care units

Delegation: assigning work to others to accomplish the work of a group

Democratic leadership style: a cooperative leadership style using ideas from the group

Developmental Theory: a mixture of physical, emotional, and social maturation and learning that an individual experiences as he or she matures

Direct delegation: involves the nurse assigning a task to another individual who is capable of performing that task but may or may not need direction and supervision

Disequilibrium: loss or lack of balance

Downsizing: streamlining organizational structure of "nonessential" positions in an effort to decrease costs

Empowerment: a person's feelings of having confidence in one's abilities

Entrepreneur: someone who takes a risk to start something new and nontraditional; often involves self-employment

Evidence-based practice: clinical interventions that are based on research

Excellence: a standard of quality that is of the highest caliber

Feasibility study: a needs assessment to determine whether it is reasonable to carry out a project or make a change

Followers: self-directing, active participants who invest themselves in fulfilling a vision that they support/endorse

Great Man Theory: one is a leader if one is born into the "right" family

Hardiness: the ability to discipline oneself to work hard; a hard work ethic

Laissez-faire leadership style: a casual leadership style that provides little direction and expects group members to lead themselves

Leadership: a process that involves articulating a vision, communicating that vision effectively, facilitating change, involving and empowering followers, holding to a standard of excellence, and creating a preferred future

Managed care: healthcare delivery system developed to decrease cost and provide comprehensive healthcare to participants who pay a standard copayment fee and use a preferred provider list

Management: a process in which a series of steps are followed to accomplish goals or implement a role within an organization structure

Mentoring: a purposeful relationship between an experienced individual and a neophyte, intended to advocate the neophyte's career

Mission: the reason for an organization's existence determines the organization's position regarding standards of practice

Negotiation: the resolution of conflict that is acceptable to the involved parties

Networking: a formation of alliances and coalitions

New Science of Leadership: a view of leadership that states that living systems organize themselves by seeking order, but this order is not linear and predictive; it implies empowerment of all, creating while doing, collaborating as a team, and evaluating process and outcomes; a moving away from a strict task focus to more of a process focused on goal accomplishment

"Once born": individuals who are very much influenced by others' opinions

Organizational culture: a way of thinking and communicating that is unique to an organization

Partnering: teamwork in which each member is equal and has similar power to make decisions

Patient outcome: result of care for a patient

Perspective Transformational: process that occurs as an individual begins to define his or her own frame of reference for nursing practice and then progresses to a clearly defined conceptual model of practice

Persuasion: being able to modify another's behavior or attitude

Philosophy: an organization's or individual's general values and beliefs

Plausible future: what is likely to occur when specific efforts are made to accomplish goals

Political astuteness: ability to influence others through political processes and strategies

Possible future: what can occur if some changes are made in the current state of affairs

Precepting: an experienced individual is assigned to guide and assist another who is learning a role

Preferred future: the future we would like to occur

Probable future: what is likely to occur when specific efforts are made to accomplish goals

Process orientation: a focus on the outcome of completing the tasks and not merely on the task completion

Quality improvement: a program that measures and tracks patient outcomes and indicators of nursing quality

Quantum Theory: specifies that interface among all group members is crucial and more significant than anything else; the world is unknowable and unpredictable

Role modeling: a method of developing and renewing others; patterning yourself after another whom you admire

Scientific Age/Industrial or Newtonian Age: emphasis on short- and long-term planning, predicting outcomes, using formulas, following bureaucratic procedures and policies, separate linear systems rather than the whole

Situational Leadership Theory: encompasses the significance of the environment and particular situation as factors in the effectiveness of a leader

Staff mix: the combination of licensed and unlicensed nursing personnel

Stewardship: holding something in trust for another; the act of serving others' interests, rather than one's own self-interests; being responsible for something more than just oneself

Strategic plan: a long-term plan consisting of how an organization plans to achieve its mission and goals

Subacute facility: a short-term facility that houses people who have been discharged from an acute-care hospital but who are not well enough to be discharged to their home or a long-term care facility

Task orientation: a focus on completing the task rather than on evaluating the outcome of the task completion

Team building: the process of learning to communicate better within a group

Team learning: the process of learning and working together in a group

Trait Theory of Leadership: implies that certain characteristics distinguish leaders from others

Trajectory: a pathway or track one follows in work, research, and/or education

Transactional leadership: both leader and followers work together to accomplish a task and generally are motivated by a financial incentive

Transformational leadership: leaders and followers work together cohesively in a highly motivated environment

"Twice born": individuals not threatened by ideas of others because their sense of self comes from within, not from their roles or expectations of others

Unlicensed assistive personnel (UAP): the workforce commonly called patient care assistants or nurse aids

Vision: dreams or ideas of a new future

Index

An "f" following a page number indicates a figure; a "t" indicates a table.